Infectious Disease PHARMACOTHERAPY *Self Assessment*

Lea S. Eiland, PharmD, BCPS, FASHP, FPPAG
Clinical Professor and Associate Department Head
Auburn University Harrison School of Pharmacy
Auburn, Alabama

Diane B. Ginsburg, PhD, RPh, FASHP
Clinical Professor
Assistant Dean for Student Affairs
College of Pharmacy
Health Outcomes and Pharmacy Practice Division
The University of Texas at Austin
Austin, Texas

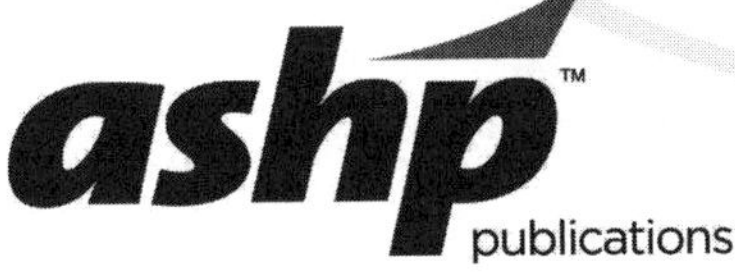

Any correspondence regarding this publication should be sent to the publisher, American Society of Health-System Pharmacists, 7272 Wisconsin Avenue, Bethesda, MD 20814, attention: Special Publishing.

Director, Special Publishing: Jack Bruggeman

Acquisitions Editor: Robin Coleman

Editorial Project Manager: Ruth Bloom

Production Manager: Kristin Eckles

Cover & Page Design: David Wade and Carol Barrer

Library of Congress Cataloging-in-Publication Data

Eiland, Lea S., author.
Infectious disease pharmacotherapy self assessment / Lea S. Eiland, Diane B. Ginsburg.
p. ; cm.
Includes bibliographical references and index.
ISBN 978-1-58528-492-4 (alk. paper)
I. Ginsburg, Diane B., author. II. American Society of Health-System Pharmacists, issuing body. III. Title.
[DNLM: 1. Communicable Diseases--drug therapy--Case Reports. 2. Communicable Diseases--drug therapy--Problems and Exercises. 3. Communicable Diseases--diagnosis--Case Reports. 4. Communicable Diseases--diagnosis--Problems and Exercises. WC 18.2]
RM301
615.1--dc23

2015012112

ISBN: 978-1-58528-492-4

10 9 8 7 6 5 4 3 2 1

DEDICATION

We dedicate this self-assessment book to those students and practitioners who participate in lifelong self-learning and strive to do better for their patients.

CONTENTS

PART I. CASES

continued on next page

CONTENTS

PART II. QUESTIONS & ANSWERS

continued on next page

CONTENTS

PREFACE

Every patient in his or her lifetime will develop an infectious disease just as pharmacists encounter infectious diseases in various populations daily. The patient may be presenting with a primary infectious disease process or with multiple problems and the added complication of an infectious process requiring specialized care and development of an appropriate treatment plan. The management of infectious diseases requires keen clinical skills and knowledge. *Infectious Disease Pharmacotherapy Self Assessment* is designed to provide clinicians with patient-specific, case-based learning for students, new practitioners, and advanced level practitioners. This textbook provides practitioners with infectious disease pharmacotherapy knowledge to care for pediatric and adult patients in various healthcare settings. Other infectious disease topics such as stewardship, antibiograms, and vaccinations are also assessed. The cases represent a range of clinical situations of varying complexity and include corresponding self-assessment questions and answers.

Each case is based on a real patient and designed to include clinical data necessary to develop a treatment plan for all aspects of care, including assessing patient-specific parameters used in the diagnosis of the infectious process; developing goals and clinical outcomes; preventing or managing comorbidities; and monitoring parameters and relevant patient/caregiver education. The intent of each case is to develop skills in identifying clinical relative patient and disease information to support a specific diagnosis and design an appropriate treatment and monitoring plan for the management of the infectious disease. The self-assessment cases may be useful for didactic coursework and preparation for both introductory and advanced pharmacy practice experiences (IPPEs/APPEs). The cases may also be valuable prior to starting a PGY1 or PGY2 residency rotation or a position focused in infectious diseases. The casebook's varying levels of difficulty allow further self-assessment after attainment of basic knowledge and skills.

The casebook is divided into two parts: patient cases (Part I) and self-assessment questions and answers (Part II). The contributors provide a variety of patient cases encountered in their respective practices. Cases are designed as level 1 (*beginner*), level 2 (*intermediate*), or level 3 (*advanced*), which allows the casebook to be a resource for students, residents, and practitioners. Sources are provided for each disease state case so that practitioners can use the primary source for additional information and/or clarification. Current practice guidelines are referenced including the CDC's *Sexually Transmitted Diseases Treatment Guidelines, 2015* and the DHHS's *Guidelines for the Use of Antiretroviral Agents in HIV-1-Infected Adults and Adolescents* (April 2015). The casebook incorporates many situations to address managing a patient with an infectious disease and handling other infectious disease issues (e.g., stewardship, infection control, etc.). The intent of the editors and contributors is to provide opportunities for self-assessment through practice and knowledge application, thereby contributing to the development of students and practitioners in managing an infectious process.

Lea S. Eiland

Diane B. Ginsburg

ACKNOWLEDGMENTS

We would like to acknowledge the following original case writers and section editors from the infectious disease section of *PharmPrep: ASHP's NAPLEX® Review, Fourth Edition*. Although cases have been changed and updated, their initial work is appreciated.

Jason Cota, PharmD, MSc
Edward H. Eiland, III, PharmD, MBA, BCPS (AQ-ID), FASHP
Lea S. Eiland, PharmD, BCPS, FASHP, FPPAG
Sharon Erdman, PharmD
John Esterly, PharmD, BCPS (AQ-ID)
Marianna Fedorenko, PharmD
Alexandria Garavaglia-Wilson, PharmD
E. Kelly Hester, PharmD, BCPS, AAHIVP
Karl Madaras-Kelly, PharmD, MPH
Catherine Oliphant, PharmD
Celtina K. Reinert, PharmD
David J. Ritchie PharmD, FCCP, BCPS (AQ-ID)
Michael P. Rivey, MS, BCPS, FASHP
Marc Scheetz, PharmD, MSc, BCPS (AQ-ID)
Amelia Sofjan, PharmD, BCPS
Collin N. Verheyden, PharmD, BCPS
Katie Vuong, PharmD
Nancy Toedter Williams, PharmD, BCPS, BCNSP, FASHP

We greatly appreciate the time and efforts of Collin N. Verheyden, PharmD, BCPS, for his review of each case. His comments and suggestions strengthened our material.

In addition, we would like to thank Edward H. Eiland, III, PharmD, MBA, BCPS (AQ-ID), FASHP, for his assistance in answering questions and providing advice about various infectious disease topics when selecting and designing each case.

Lastly, a sincere thank-you to the ASHP Special Publications staff who listened to our ideas and assisted in the development of this self-assessment textbook. We are proud to be part of the self-assessment series to assist students and practitioners in strengthening their patient care knowledge related to infectious diseases.

PART 1 | CASES

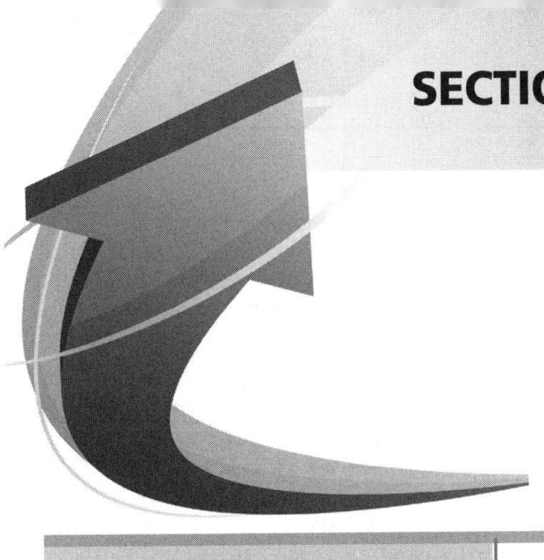

CASE 1.1
Acute Osteomyelitis | Level 1

Demographics

Patient Name: Michael Thomas

Age: 18

Sex: Male

Height: 5′8″

Weight: 150 lb

Race: Caucasian

Allergies: NKDA

Chief Complaint: M. T. presents to the ED complaining that his left arm is hurting and swollen.

History of Present Illness: M. T. broke his left radius playing soccer 14 days ago. He required surgery and placement of a metal plate to hold the bones in place. He states that all has been well until yesterday when he bumped his arm on a door frame. A few hours later, he noticed the swelling, and it has gotten worse with increasing pain.

Review of Systems: Left arm is notably swollen, red, and hot to the touch; no other systems reviewed

Past Medical History: Past medical history is unremarkable except for normal childhood illnesses.

Social History: M. T. is a high school senior who lives at home with his sister, brother, mother, and father. He is very active physically. He denies drinking alcohol and using tobacco products or other illicit drugs.

Family History: Mother—seasonal allergies; father—HTN; brother—asthma

Medications: Hydrocodone/acetaminophen 5 mg/500 mg 1 tablet po q 6 hr prn pain postsurgery

Physical Examination

Gen: Alert and oriented; cooperative, pleasant, and animated in conversation

VS: Ht 5′8″, Wt 150 lb, HR 77 bpm, RR 19 rpm, T 101.8°F, BP 122/75 mm Hg

HEENT: Unremarkable

Chest: Lungs CTA, heart RRR

Abd: Soft, nondistended

Neuro: Not checked

Laboratory and Diagnostic Tests

CBC: WBC 16,200 no differential

ESR: 80 mm/hr

CRP: 12 mg/dL

X-ray: Possible but not definitive blurring of margins of left radius at point of fracture

Technetium Bone Scan: Positive for inflammation in the left radius

Blood Cultures: Pending

Diagnosis

Acute osteomyelitis

Notes

The orthopedic surgeon is consulted to determine if surgical debridement is needed.

SELF-ASSESSMENT QUESTIONS

1. What are the clinical findings of osteomyelitis and what are potential complications of the disease?
2. What is the most likely microbiologic etiology for the suspected osteomyelitis?
3. M. T. appears very agitated and preoccupied on initial presentation to the emergency department. He explains that he has tickets to a sold-out concert for that evening and was hoping to get a "shot of some kind" and then be sent home with oral antibiotics. His classmate was recently prescribed oral ciprofloxacin for a wound infection, and he was hoping to get a similar prescription. Which of the following counseling points regarding treatment of his osteomyelitis is ***not*** correct?
   a. Only parenteral antibiotics are used in the management of osteomyelitis.
   b. Antibiotics used in the treatment of osteomyelitis generally are given in high doses.
   c. Early antibiotic therapy may reduce the need for surgery.
   d. Ciprofloxacin has poor activity against staphylococci and would not be a good initial antibiotic choice for him.
   e. The duration of antibiotic therapy for osteomyelitis is usually 4 to 6 weeks.
4. M. T. is initiated on vancomycin but does not tolerate it, so the physician decides to change to a different parenteral antibiotic regimen. After consulting with the pharmacist, either linezolid or daptomycin is recommended as an alternative option. Which one of the following statements is ***not*** correct regarding IV linezolid and daptomycin therapies?
   a. Selective serotonin reuptake inhibitors (SSRIs), such as fluoxetine, may cause a serotonin syndrome when administered with linezolid.
   b. Thrombocytopenia is a recognized adverse effect of linezolid.
   c. Concurrent ingestion of large amounts of tyramine-containing foods, such as aged or matured cheese, with daptomycin may cause sudden and severe high blood pressure.
   d. Creatine kinase concentrations should be monitored at least weekly during daptomycin therapy.
   e. Concurrent administration of HMG-CoA reductase inhibitors with daptomycin may increase the risk of myopathies.
5. After receiving 7 days of parenteral antibiotics, the physician decides to switch M. T. to oral therapy. His strain of methicillin-resistant *Staphylococcus aureus* (MRSA) is sensitive to all the expected antibiotics. Which are the options for treating his infection?
6. Approximately 2 weeks after switching to oral therapy (3 weeks total of oral and parenteral antibiotics), the patient visits you and states a desire to discontinue his antibiotic. He explains that at his last doctor's appointment 2 days ago, the physician told him that he had no fever, his WBC count was back to normal, and the physical exam was unremarkable with no swelling, redness, or tenderness at the surgical wound site. How would you counsel this patient?

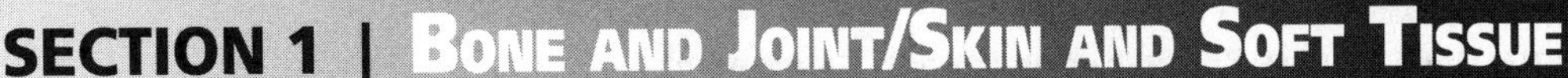

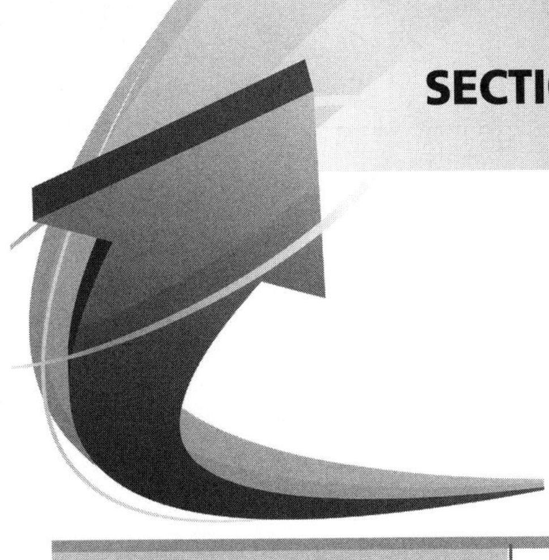

CASE 1.2
Skin and Soft Tissue Infection | Level 2

Demographics

PATIENT NAME: Don Hamilton

AGE: 58

SEX: Male

HEIGHT: 6′2″

WEIGHT: 76.1 kg

RACE: Caucasian

ALLERGIES: NKDA

CHIEF COMPLAINT: D. H., a 58-year-old male, presents to the ED with complaints of a reddened, swollen, and painful right knee after striking it on a tree while snowmobiling.

HISTORY OF PRESENT ILLNESS: D. H. was in his usual state of health until about a week ago when he went snowmobiling and accidentally bumped his knee on a tree. Later that day he went swimming in a natural hot springs. The next day he noticed an ingrown hair with a small blackened blister around the hair follicle. Over the following day, the area surrounding the follicle became more erythematous and painful. He was seen in a clinic and prescribed cephalexin 500 mg po qid for 7 days. Three days after starting the cephalexin, there was a silver-dollar sized scab and three new blister-like lesions that were fluctuant on his knee, and his leg was erythematous and edematous. He was seen in clinic a second time, and one of the blister-like lesions was incised and drained. A small amount of pus was sent to the lab for culture, and he was prescribed dicloxacillin 250 mg po qid for 10 days. Two days after starting the dicloxacillin, D. H. noticed the edema and erythema moving up his leg to his mid-thigh over the weekend and drove to the ED for further evaluation. The culture obtained 2 days ago is growing 4+ coagulase-positive *Staphylococcus*.

REVIEW OF SYSTEMS: Complains of chills, feeling fatigued, and 7 out of 10 pain in lower right leg

PAST MEDICAL HISTORY: Peptic ulcer disease with history of *H. Pylori* (treated with triple therapy); osteoarthritis; bilateral arthroscopic knee surgery (1998); hyperlipidemia; left partial kidney resection due to complicated cyst

Social History: Lives out of town with second wife, has three grown children, and is retired from the Air Force where he worked in a missile silo; no tobacco, occasional alcohol, no illicit drug use

Family History: Father—died at age 72 of MI; mother and all siblings—alive

Physical Examination

Gen: NAD, well-nourished male

VS: T 102.7°F, BP 121/73 mm Hg, HR 90 bpm, RR 20 rpm

HEENT: NC/AT, EOMI, PERRLA, OP clear, mucous membranes moist, no LAD or masses; normocephalic, atraumatic

Lungs: CTAB, no wheezes or crackles

CV: RRR, normal S1/S2; no m/r/g

Abd: Soft, no organomegaly, no masses or tenderness, normal BS

Neuro: CN II-XII grossly intact; 5/5 upper and lower extremity strength; negative Romberg

Ext: 90° flexion only on right knee; full ROM all other joints; no tenderness to palpation in calf

Skin: Several blackened blister-like lesions varying in size from 5–15 cm surrounding 20-cm macerated skin gouge distal to the right knee; entire knee erythematous and edematous; erythema to mid-calf and mid-thigh

Laboratory and Diagnostic Tests

Obtained in ED on Day of Admission

Sodium: 142 mEq/L

Potassium: 3.9 mEq/L

Chloride: 108 mEq/L

CO_2 Content: 26 mmol/L

BUN: 18 mg/dL

Serum Creatinine: 1.1 mg/dL

Glucose: 94 mg/dL

WBC: 12.4 K/μL

RBC: 5.07 m/μL

Hemoglobin: 15.1 g/dL

Hematocrit: 45.0%

Platelets: 345 K/μL

Neut%: 70.2

Lymph%: 12.6

Mono%: 9.8

Eos%: 1.2

Baso%: 0.2

Bands%: 6

Microbiology

Specimen source: aspirate from fluctuant lesion, 2 days prior

Coagulase-positive *Staphylococcus aureus*

Susceptibility

ampicillin/sulbactam R

cefazolin R

ceftriaxone R

ciprofloxacin R

clindamycin S

daptomycin S

erythromycin R

linezolid S

oxacillin R

trimethoprim/sulfamethoxazole S

tetracycline S

vancomycin S (MIC = 1 mcg/mL)

Diagnosis

Skin and soft tissue infection

Medication Record

Home Medications

Simvastatin 40 mg qhs

Acetaminophen 1,000 mg po tid

Maalox 15 mL prn heartburn

Started 5 days ago: Cephalexin 500 mg 1 po qid × 7 days

Started 2 days ago: Dicloxacillin 250 mg po qid × 10 days

Hospital Course

Vancomycin 1 g IV q 12 hr and piperacillin/tazobactam 3.375 g IV q 8 hr started for empirical coverage of severe cellulitis of unknown origin not responsive to gram-positive coverage with beta-lactam antibiotics; renal function normal; vancomycin trough ordered post 4th dose

Hydrocodone/acetaminophen 5/500 mg 1–2 tablets po q 4–6 hr prn initiated

SELF-ASSESSMENT QUESTIONS

1. Name the organisms that are a common cause for the following:
   a. Uncomplicated nonpurulent cellulitis
   b. Skin infections involving furuncles, carbuncles, or abscesses
2. What are the risk factors for methicillin-resistant *S. aureus* (MRSA) infections, and which oral antibiotics can be used to treat community-acquired MRSA (CA-MRSA) skin infections as an outpatient?
3. D. H. was placed on vancomycin intravenously for his CA-MRSA. The pharmacist is responsible for adjusting the dose based on levels. After four doses at 1,000 mg IV every 12 hours, his serum trough vancomycin level is 4.5 mg/dL. What should the pharmacist do regarding his vancomycin dose and regimen?
4. What if the susceptibility test showed the vancomycin MIC returned as 2 mcg/mL? What should the pharmacist do regarding his vancomycin dose and regimen?
5. In the hospital, D. H. is placed in contact isolation due to his MRSA infection in an attempt to prevent other patients from becoming infected. What infection control procedures are necessary while D. H. is in the hospital?
6. In which of the following skin infections is topical antibiotic therapy most appropriate?
   a. Cellulitis in a healthy adult female
   b. Impetigo in a teenager
   c. Erysipelas with associated fever and chills
   d. Deep bite wound received by a human
   e. Diabetic foot infection
7. What if D. H. presents to the ED with only a cut on the bottom of his foot that looks infected? He has fever, chills, and an elevated WBC count. He states that 2 days ago he stepped on a piece of broken glass at the bottom of a swimming pool and that the glass cut his foot. The physician wants to prescribe cephalexin as empiric treatment for this skin and soft tissue infection. What should the pharmacist say?
   a. Infections that occur in under-chlorinated swimming pools or hot tubs can be caused by *Pseudomonas aeruginosa*. Cephalexin does not possess activity against *P. aeruginosa*, and the patient should receive oral ciprofloxacin.
   b. Infections that occur in under-chlorinated swimming pools or hot tubs can be caused by *P. aeruginosa*, which has high intrinsic resistance to all oral cephalosporins, and moxifloxacin should be used to treat the infection.
   c. This foot infection is likely caused by a food and water contaminant like *Shigella* or *Salmonella* and should be treated with oral trimethoprim/sulfamethoxazole.
   d. This foot infection is likely caused by *Streptococcus pyogenes*, a common cause of cellulitis. Cephalexin is an excellent choice, and I will fill the prescription right away.
   e. Ertapenem should be prescribed rather than cephalexin to cover for likely pathogens including *P. aeruginosa*.

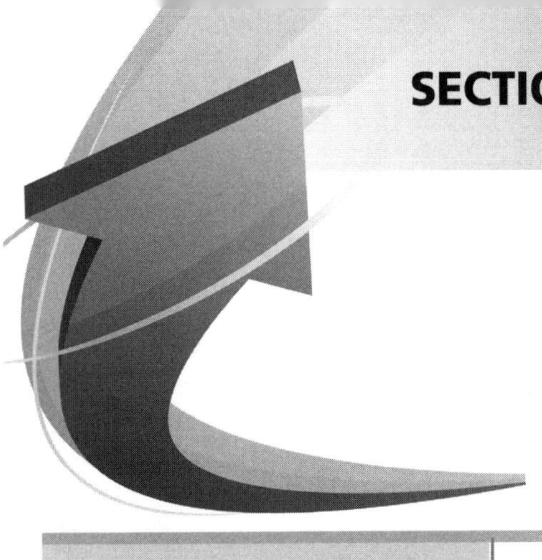

CASE 1.3
Diabetic Foot Infection | Level 3

Demographics

Patient Name: John Taylor

Age: 72

Sex: Male

Height: 6′1″

Weight: 165 lb

Race: African American

Allergies: Sulfa (hives)

Chief Complaint: J. T.'s wife brings him to the ED because "his foot looks infected."

History of Present Illness: J. T.'s wife noticed his socks were discolored for the past week when she was washing clothes. She asked him if something was wrong, but he denied any issues. Today, she noticed his feet smelled funny, and when she removed his sock, she noticed a crack in his foot and pus coming from it. Upon further questioning, J. T. states he has had no issues and is here only to make his wife happy.

Review of Systems: Right foot is notably swollen, red, and hot to the touch; no other systems reviewed

Past Medical History: Type 2 diabetes mellitus; HTN; hyperlipidemia

Social History: Smoked 1 pack per day for 20 years, quit 25 years ago; denies alcohol or illicit drug use; attends water aerobics three times a week

Family History: Mother—died from stroke at age 65; father—HTN; brother—type 2 diabetes mellitus

Immunization History: Up-to-date

Physical Examination

Gen: Alert and oriented; cooperative but not wanting to be in the ED

VS: Ht 6′1″, Wt 165 lb, HR 77 bpm, RR 19 rpm, T 100.8°F, BP 124/77 mm Hg

HEENT: Unremarkable

CHEST: Lungs CTA, heart RRR

ABD: Soft, nondistended

NEURO: Numbness in both feet, up to the calf (did not respond to microfilament testing)

EXT: Ulcer on bottom of right foot, 2+ edema, erythematous, draining yellowish pus, wound probe about 1-cm deep, normal range of motion, pedal pulses present

Laboratory and Diagnostic Tests

SODIUM: 138 mEq/L

POTASSIUM: 4.1 mEq/L

CHLORIDE: 102 mEq/L

CO_2 CONTENT: 25 mEq/L

BUN: 20 mg/dL

SERUM CREATININE: 1.2 mg/dL

GLUCOSE: 220 mg/dL

HEMOGLOBIN: 14.3 g/dL

HEMATOCRIT: 44%

PLATELETS: 350,000 cells/mm^3

A1C: 9%

CBC: WBC 14,200 cells/mm^3, 80% PMNs, 5% bands

ESR: 85 mm/hr

CRP: 7 mg/dL

X-RAY: Significant tissue destruction, no abscess noted, cannot determine bony involvement

TECHNETIUM BONE SCAN: Negative for inflammation in the right foot

WOUND AND BLOOD CULTURES: Pending

Diagnosis

Diabetic foot infection

Medication Record

Pravastatin 20 mg po daily

Glyburide/metformin 5 mg/500 mg 1 tablet po bid

Lisinopril 20 mg po daily

SELF-ASSESSMENT QUESTIONS

1. What is the most likely microbiologic etiology for a diabetic foot infection?
2. Based on the *2012 Infectious Diseases Society of America Clinical Practice Guideline for the Diagnosis and Treatment of Diabetic Foot Infections*, what is the classification of this diabetic foot infection?
3. Develop an empiric treatment plan for J. T.
4. J. T.'s blood cultures report no growth, and his wound cultures report positive for *Pseudomonas aeruginosa* and *Bacteroides fragilis*. Susceptibilities are listed below:

P. aeruginosa	
Cefepime	I
Ciprofloxacin	R
Gentamicin	S
Imipenem/cilastatin	S
Piperacillin/tazobactam	S
Tobramycin	S

   B. fragilis: No susceptibility report provided

   What alterations, if any, would you recommend for your treatment plan?
5. You are asked to be the pharmacist member on a new antimicrobial stewardship team. The team is deciding how to measure adult antibiotic use in the inpatient setting. What do you suggest the team uses for metrics?
6. What if J. T. had presented with a mild diabetic foot infection and the wound culture grew MRSA? What would be the treatment regimen and duration?

CASE 1.4

Gastrointestinal Infection—*Clostridium difficile* | Level 1

Demographics

PATIENT NAME: James Worthington

AGE: 42

SEX: Male

HEIGHT: 6′0″

WEIGHT: 180 lb

RACE: White

ALLERGIES: Azithromycin (skin rash)

CHIEF COMPLAINT: J. W. is a 42-year-old man who presents to the ED with a 3- to 4-day history of diarrhea and intermittent abdominal pain and cramping.

HISTORY OF PRESENT ILLNESS: J. W. and his family have been vacationing for the past week out-of-state in the region. His diarrhea had its onset 3 days ago and has worsened. Although he reports four to six bowel movements daily during that time, he suffers from urgency and reports the feeling he "has to sit on the toilet all day." Stools have been watery until this morning, when he passed a mucous, blood-tinged stool. He has taken two tablets of Imodium for each of the past 2 days, which slowed the diarrhea and allowed him to attend work. His illness has been associated with fatigue, occasional chills, and intermittent lower left abdominal pain and cramping. He reports no change in his appetite or weight and no night sweats since the onset of his illness. He presents to the ED concerned about the bloody stool. Just before his vacation, he finished a 10-day course of cefuroxime axetil that he received for a painful sore throat with laryngitis and cough productive of a greenish sputum. J. W. believes the diarrhea is related to the antibiotic use, despite his use of probiotics.

REVIEW OF SYSTEMS: Otherwise noncontributory

PAST MEDICAL HISTORY: No history of diverticulitis or constipation; appendectomy 15 years ago, without complications

SOCIAL HISTORY: Married with a 10-year-old son; healthy wife and son without current illness; denies tobacco or drug use; estimates 3 alcoholic drinks per month

Family History: Healthy parents in their 70s (mother had a colonic polyp removed a few years ago); no history of colon cancer or inflammatory bowel disease in the family

Physical Examination

Gen: Alert, oriented white male comfortable in NAD; appears slightly thin

VS: Afebrile T 97.8°F, BP 131/72 mm Hg, HR 79 bpm, RR 16 rpm, Wt 180 lb, Ht 6′0″

HEENT: PERRLA, unremarkable

Neck: Supple with normal ROM

Chest: Clear to auscultation

CV: Regular rhythm

Abd: Flat, soft, with present BS diminished; tenderness only to very deep palpation in left lower quadrant; no guarding or rebound; no masses or peritoneal signs; no CVAT

Rect: Small hemorrhoid that is not swollen, not tender, and without bright red blood present; no stool on exam; no tenderness noted

Laboratory and Diagnostic Tests

WBC: 9,700 cells/mm^3 with 75% PMNs, 13% lymphocytes, 11% monocytes, 1% basophils

Hemoglobin: 15.5 g/dL

Hematocrit: 45.6%

Platelets: 158,000 cells/mm^3

Sodium: 144 mEq/L

Potassium: 4.0 mEq/L

Chloride: 103 mEq/L

CO_2 Content: 26 mEq/L

Serum Creatinine: 0.8 mg/dL

BUN: 10 mg/dL

Glucose: 98 mg/dL

Calcium: 9.2 mg/dL

Pulse Oximetry: 98% on room air

Stool Analysis: (+) occult blood, moderate WBCs

Stool Culture: (–) *Salmonella, Shigella, Campylobacter, E. coli* 0157, *Yersinia, Aeromonas, Plesiomonas*; no significant number of *Candida*; (+) *Clostridium difficile* (*C. difficile*) toxin A and/or B

Diagnosis

C. difficile infection (CDI)

SELF-ASSESSMENT QUESTIONS

1. Develop a pharmacologic plan for the treatment of the CDI.
2. Which one of the following statements is ***true*** regarding *C. difficile* enterocolitis testing and diagnosis?
   a. *C. difficile* enterocolitis is typically diagnosed in clinical settings by isolation of the organism from the stool.
   b. Isolation of the *C. difficile* organism is rare in neonates or infants.
   c. False-negative testing results for *C. difficile* are common.
   d. The majority of patients in whom the *C. difficile* organism could be isolated will remain asymptomatic for diarrhea.
   e. Laboratory testing for *C. difficile* is recommended in all ICU patients because outbreaks commonly occur in this setting.
3. Name at least three risk factors for developing a CDI.
4. Which of the following statements is ***true*** regarding metronidazole (Flagyl) treatment of *C. difficile* enterocolitis?
   a. The drug is effective only if given by the oral route of administration.
   b. Relapse rate following a course of metronidazole is less than 2%.
   c. The drug is an appropriate first choice in patients of all conditions and ages with *C. difficile* enterocolitis.
   d. The failure rate for metronidazole treatment of *C. difficile* enterocolitis appears to be increasing.
   e. A 3- to 5-day course of metronidazole therapy may be used in patients presenting with mild *C. difficile* enterocolitis.

5. A medical resident asks you when vancomycin should be used as an appropriate alternative to metronidazole for *C. difficile* enterocolitis. Vancomycin should be considered for therapy in all ***except*** which one of the following patient types?
   a. The patient is intolerant to metronidazole.
   b. The patient has failed to respond to an adequate course of metronidazole.
   c. The patient has gastrointestinal tract complications and must be treated with IV drug therapy.
   d. The patient has severe, life-threatening *C. difficile* enterocolitis.
   e. The patient is suffering a second recurrence of *C. difficile* enterocolitis.

6. Which of the following statements is ***true*** regarding options for the treatment of *C. difficile* enterocolitis?
   a. Treatment with recommended pharmacotherapeutic agents is always required when *C. difficile* enterocolitis is diagnosed.
   b. Fidaxomicin is a newer treatment option that is superior in efficacy to vancomycin for treatment of an initial episode of *C. difficile* enterocolitis.
   c. Fidaxomicin has been proven to be a cost-effective treatment for all patients with recurrent *C. difficile* enterocolitis.
   d. Probiotics have been proven to help prevent *C. difficile* enterocolitis when added to antimicrobial therapy.
   e. Combination therapy with oral vancomycin plus IV metronidazole is recommended for initial treatment of severe, complicated *C. difficile* enterocolitis.

CASE 1.5
Gastrointestinal Infection—*Shigella* | Level 2

Demographics

PATIENT NAME: Trevor Knight

AGE: 9

SEX: Male

HEIGHT: 4′6″

WEIGHT: 64 lb

RACE: White

ALLERGIES: NKDA

CHIEF COMPLAINT: T. K. is a 9-year-old child brought to the ED by his mother with a 3-day history of diarrhea with severe abdominal cramping and pain, fever, and malaise.

HISTORY OF PRESENT ILLNESS: T. K. is an avid young fisherman who returned earlier in the week from a backpacking and fishing trip with his father in Yellowstone National Park. They hiked through primitive areas without sanitation and camped in sites commonly used by other hikers. He states he started to feel poorly 5 days ago, which was the day after the trip concluded. His parents noted his illness 3 days ago when he developed a fever and watery diarrhea with cramping, but he continued to eat and drink in his usual amount. His mother encouraged additional fluid intake for his diarrhea and gave him acetaminophen for his fevers, which were sporadic. He was not given any antidiarrheal medication. His mother believes his diarrhea seemed to worsen over the next 24 to 48 hours, but she says it has lessened over the past 24 hours. She notes continued malaise in the child and states that he now looks "sicker" than when the diarrhea started. The child has continued to complain of abdominal pain throughout the illness. Today he noticed his stools contained blood and mucus, which was confirmed by his parents, who decided to bring him to the clinic. His mother also notes increasing lethargy in the child in the past 24 hours.

REVIEW OF SYSTEMS: Otherwise noncontributory

PAST MEDICAL HISTORY: Noncontributory; no serious diseases other than a few typical childhood otitis media and upper respiratory infections; no serious injury

SOCIAL HISTORY: Lives with his parents and three sisters, ages 2, 4, and 6

Family History: Father—age 39, controlled hyperlipidemia; mother—age 36 years, healthy; two sisters—healthy; grandfather—died of a heart attack at age 64; other grandparents —healthy; no known history of cancer or diabetes in family

Immunization History: Up-to-date

Physical Examination

Gen: Juvenile white male is oriented, alert, and cooperative to exam but clearly lethargic. He appears to be in moderate distress and complains of abdominal pain. Color is somewhat pale, and he appears to be mildly-to-moderately dehydrated.

VS: T 102.3°F taken orally, RR 20 rpm, BP 124/78 mm Hg, HR 72 bpm, Wt 64 lb

HEENT: Oral mucous membranes are dry, PERRLA, otherwise unremarkable

Neck: Supple without masses

Chest: Lungs CTA; cardiovascular: normal rate and rhythm

Abd: BS increased in all quadrants; diffuse tenderness; no masses appreciated; no rebound tenderness; no evidence for peritonitis; patient does guard on palpation but rigidity not present

Neuro: Reflexes equal and symmetrical; motor strength normal

Rect: External exam only; normal findings with no fissures

Skin: Slight loss of color consistent with some dehydration

Laboratory and Diagnostic Tests

Sodium: 135 mEq/L

Potassium: 3.8 mEq/L

Chloride: 98 mEq/L

CO_2 Content: 22 mEq/L

Glucose: 120 mg/dL

BUN: 18 mg/dL

Serum Creatinine: 0.5 mg/dL

AST: 25 international units/L

ALT: 22 international units/L

INR: 1.0

WBC: 10,300 cells/mm^3 with 85% PMNs, 8% lymphocytes, 5% monocytes, 2% eosinophils

Hemoglobin: 14.3 g/dL

Hematocrit: 40.9%

Platelets: 305,000 cells/mm^3

Stool Analysis: Watery, red-brown in color with mucus in appearance, (+) for occult blood and WBCs

Stool Culture: Positive for *Shigella sonnei*; negative for *Salmonella*, *Campylobacter*, and *E. coli* serotype 0157, ova and parasites, and *C. difficile* toxin

Diagnosis

Shigella gastroenteritis (GE)

Medication Record

Acetaminophen 2 tsp po q 4–6 hr prn

SELF-ASSESSMENT QUESTIONS

1. All ***except*** which one of the following characteristics helped to distinguish bacterial from viral GE in T. K.?
   a. Recovery of fecal leukocytes from the stool is common in bacterial GE but rare in viral GE.
   b. Bloody diarrhea is common in bacterial GE but rare in viral GE.
   c. Travel-related GE can be caused by either bacterial or viral pathogens.
   d. Elements of dehydration were present in T. K., and those rarely occur with viral GE.
   e. Temperature elevations (fevers) are typically more elevated in bacterial compared to viral GE.
2. What is the most common pathogen in acute GE in children less than 10 years of age?
3. What was the most important risk factor for the development of shigellosis in T. K.?

4. Which antimicrobial agent is preferred in current pediatric guidelines as the treatment of choice of shigellosis?
5. All ***except*** which one of the following statements are true regarding *Shigella* GE in the entire population?
   a. Shigellosis is commonly a self-limited disease that does not require antimicrobial therapy.
   b. *Shigella sonnei* is the most common cause of shigellosis in the United States.
   c. Shigellosis in the United States most commonly occurs in adult patients.
   d. Shigellosis is diagnosed by the isolation of the organism in a stool culture.
   e. *Shigella* has no natural reservoir in nature and is passed from person to person.
6. What type of medication is not recommended for patients like T. K. who suffer from bloody diarrhea and dehydration in association with shigellosis?

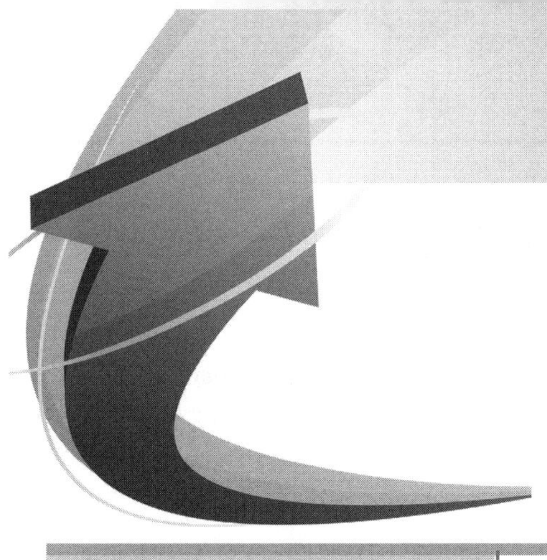

CASE 1.6
Meningitis | Level 2

Demographics

PATIENT NAME: Tony Depp

AGE: 22

SEX: Male

HEIGHT: 6′2″

WEIGHT: 210 lb

RACE: White

ALLERGIES: Sulfa (rash)

CHIEF COMPLAINT: "I have the worst headache of my life."

HISTORY OF PRESENT ILLNESS: T. D. is a 22-year-old college senior who was brought to the ED by his girlfriend on 10/20 due to decreased energy, general malaise, and an excruciating headache since last night. His symptoms were of sudden onset and have persisted about 6 hours. The patient attended a party the night of the onset of symptoms. He denies illicit drug use but did consume 5 cans of beer prior to the development of symptoms. On admission to the ED, the patient continues to complain about headache, sensitivity to light, and neck stiffness. The patient has vomited once since presenting to the ED and is continually nauseated.

REVIEW OF SYSTEMS: Exam reveals an ill-appearing young male who is only able to respond to questions intermittently with "yes/no" answers but denies any focal pain. The patient appears somnolent but is arousable.

PAST MEDICAL HISTORY: T. D. has a past medical history of seasonal allergies as well as intermittent insomnia.

SOCIAL HISTORY: Travel history—during summer, backpacked across Western Europe (France, Germany, Spain, and Italy); tobacco use—social smoker (approximately 1 pack every 2 weeks), began smoking at the age of 16; alcohol use—approximately 12 drinks per week (mainly on weekends); recreational drug use—denied by patient and girlfriend; caffeine use—2 cups of coffee per day (use is doubled during exams); lives in apartment with two other male roommates

FAMILY HISTORY: Father—50-year-old male alive and well with hypothyroidism; mother—51-year-old female alive and well with no known medical problems

Vaccination History: Influenza vaccine—receives annually; childhood series—up-to-date

Physical Examination

Gen: Pale, well-nourished, lethargic male in NAD

VS: On ED admission, BP 110/68 mm Hg, HR 120 bpm, RR 22 rpm, T 102°F, Ht 6′2″, Wt 210 lb

HEENT: No papilledema on exam; pupils equally round and reactive to light; patient with photophobia

Chest: Clear to auscultation

CV: RRR with normal S1/S2 and no audible murmur

Neuro: Intermittently alert; oriented to self (patient is unable to state where he is or what day it is); nuchal rigidity present, positive Brudzinski's sign, positive Kernig's sign

Ext: Notable for several petechial skin lesions on arms

Skin: Petechiae present as noted below

Laboratory and Diagnostic Tests

Sodium: 140 mEq/L

Potassium: 4 mEq/L

Chloride: 106 mEq/L

CO_2 Content: 28 mEq/L

BUN: 30 mg/dL

Serum Creatinine: 1.3 mg/dL

Glucose: 106 mg/dL

Hemoglobin: 16.2 g/dL

Hematocrit: 49%

Platelets: 281,000 cells/mm^3

WBC: 20,600 cells/mm^3 with 75% PMNs, 18% bands, 3% lymphocytes, 4% monocytes

Blood Toxicology/Alcohol Screen: Negative

Head CT: Normal

CXR: Normal

Lumbar Puncture/CSF: WBC 2,700 cells/mm^3, 88% segs, 6% lymphocytes, 6% monocytes, 10 RBCs, glucose 7 mg/dL, protein 610 mg/dL

CSF Gram Stain: Gram-negative diplococci

Diagnosis

Meningitis

Medication Record

Home Medications

Fluticasone 50 mcg, 1 spray per nostril daily

Zolpidem 10 mg, 1 tablet prn insomnia

SELF-ASSESSMENT QUESTIONS

1. Name two organisms that are the most likely pathogens in our 22-year-old immunocompetent patient with suspected community-acquired meningitis.
2. Which anti-infectives would provide optimal (yet the most narrow spectrum) empiric coverage for meningitis prior to microbiology laboratory findings in this patient?
3. After 3 days of therapy, the pathogen is determined to be *Neisseria meningitidis*. Which statement most accurately summarizes the utility of corticosteroids in this patient?
    a. Dexamethasone should be initiated in this patient because the culture confirmed *N. meningitidis*.
    b. Dexamethasone should be initiated in this patient to decrease inflammation associated with concomitant enterovirus infection.
    c. Dexamethasone should have been initiated early in this patient, but delay in therapy and uncertain efficacy of dexamethasone in *N. meningitidis* precludes its current utility at this point in the clinical course.
    d. Because the culture confirmed *N. meningitidis*, dexamethasone should not be initiated in this patient as it will decrease the penetration of vancomycin, and vancomycin will be unable to treat the *N. meningitidis*.

e. Dexamethasone should not be initiated in this patient due to the patient's leukocytosis. This is a black box warning and an absolute contraindication.

4. What are the prophylaxis regimen options for household contacts of a patient diagnosed with community-acquired meningitis caused by *N. meningitidis*? Does his girlfriend warrant prophylaxis?

5. T. D. has been in close contact with his sister, who is currently 8 months pregnant, and her physician wants to initiate chemoprophylaxis. Which chemoprophylaxis regimen should she receive?

6. Which populations does the Advisory Committee on Immunization Practices (ACIP) currently recommend receiving routine administration of the *N. meningitidis* vaccine?

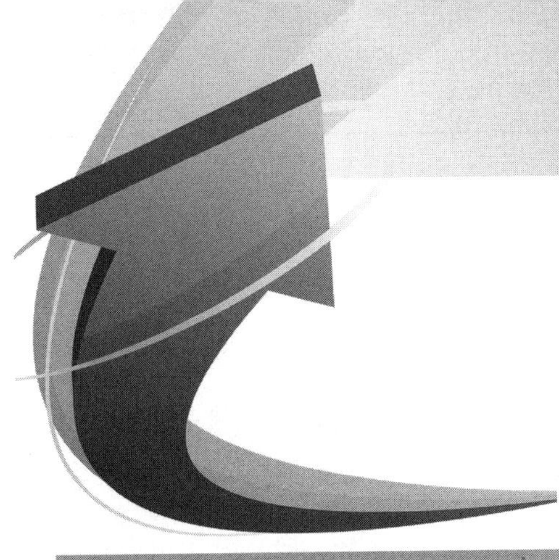

CASE 1.7
Neurosyphilis | Level 3

Demographics

Patient Name: Greg Jefferies

Age: 50

Sex: Male

Height: 6′4″

Weight: 233 lb

Race: White

Allergies: Penicillin (anaphylaxis)

Chief Complaint: G. J. is a 50-year-old white male who is admitted to the hospital for treatment of asymptomatic neurosyphilis. G. J. is without complaints and reports no manifestations of infection. Presence of infection was identified when a routine screening test, conducted in conjunction with application for a marriage license, was positive for syphilis rapid plasma reagin antibody. Follow-up specific treponemal tests of serum and CSF confirmed the presence of infection.

History of Present Illness: G. J. reports no complaints at present. He notes that he received treatment with unknown antibiotics 7 years ago for an STD that he acquired during "a period of sexual indiscretion" following his divorce. At that time, he presented with dysuria and a purulent urethral discharge and was informed that he had gonorrhea. He noted at that time that the infection was most likely acquired from one of several one-night encounters with women he had met in a bar. He was unable to identify the index source, so follow-up and treatment of the reference case did not occur. Following treatment, he reports rapid resolution of symptoms and no subsequent sequela. He denies observing the occurrence of any manifestations or symptoms suggestive of syphilis following this course of treatment.

Review of Systems: Normal

Past Medical History: G. J. has a history of HTN that is currently controlled and a history of STD exposure as noted above. He also reports a history of a severe allergic reaction to penicillin. He notes that 23 years ago, he received a prescription for penicillin for treatment of a sore throat. Immediately after taking the first dose, he noted shortness of breath accompanied by swelling of his face, neck, and tongue. He was rushed to the ED, where he received a "shot of adrenaline" and was observed until symptoms abated. He was informed at that time that he should avoid penicillin or all penicillin-like antibiotics in the future. The remainder of his history is unremarkable and is noncontributory.

Social History: G. J. has been divorced from his first wife for 8 years and has been involved in a monogamous relationship with his current partner, to whom he is engaged, for the last 2 years. He reports that he used condoms with all his sexual contacts following diagnosis and treatment of the STD 7 years ago up to his current partner. He reports that he and his fiancé quit using condoms about 3 months into their relationship. Tobacco use—chewing tobacco, 2 cans per week; alcohol use—3 to 4 beers or glasses of wine per week; caffeine use—3 to 4 cups of decaffeinated coffee per day.

Family History: Father—died in an MVA at age 58; mother—alive at age 72; two brothers—ages 58 and 52; one sister—age 44; three children—ages 26, 24, and 19

Physical Examination

Gen: Well-nourished, white male in NAD

VS: BP 134/82 mm Hg, HR 72 bpm, RR 20 rpm, T 37.5°C, Ht 6′4″, Wt 106 kg

HEENT: Normal, no adenopathy palpable

Lungs: Clear breath sounds

CV: RRR with normal S1/S2 and no audible murmur

Skin: No erythema or petechiae

GU: Normal

Neuro: Alert and oriented; normal reflexes elicited and normal gait observed

Laboratory and Diagnostic Tests

Sodium: 144 mEq/L

Potassium: 4.5 mEq/L

Chloride: 103 mEq/L

CO_2 Content: 22 mEq/L

BUN: 25 mg/dL

Serum Creatinine: 1.2 mg/dL

Glucose: 110 mg/dL

Hemoglobin: 12.4 g/dL

Hematocrit: 37%

Platelets: 385,000 cells/mm^3

WBC: 5,600 cells/mm^3 with 75% PMNs, 20% lymphocytes, 4% monocytes, 1% eosinophils

Serum: RPR-1:256, FTA-ABS-reactive

CSF: VDRL-1:32

Diagnosis

Neurosyphilis

Medication Record

Amlodipine 5 mg po daily

SELF-ASSESSMENT QUESTIONS

1. What is the most appropriate treatment (drug and regimen) for the following:
   a. Neurosyphilis
   b. Primary syphilis
   c. Primary syphilis in a penicillin-allergic patient
2. What are characteristic findings of primary, secondary, and tertiary neurosyphilis?
3. G. J. is initiated on treatment and calls the nurse later that afternoon with complaints of fever, headache, and sore muscles. What is the best recommendation for G. J.?
4. What is the drug of choice for the treatment of syphilis in a pregnant patient with a penicillin allergy?
5. In monitoring a patient for the treatment of syphilis, what lab change would indicate efficacy of treatment?
6. What combination of labs and clinical disease meets the definition of latent syphilis?
   a. (+) RPR, (–) FTA-ABS, (–) clinical disease
   b. (+) RPR, (+) FTA-ABS, (+) clinical disease
   c. (+) RPR, (+) FTA-ABS, (–) clinical disease
   d. (–) RPR, (+) FTA-ABS, (+) clinical disease
   e. (+) RPR, (–) FTA-ABS, (+) clinical disease

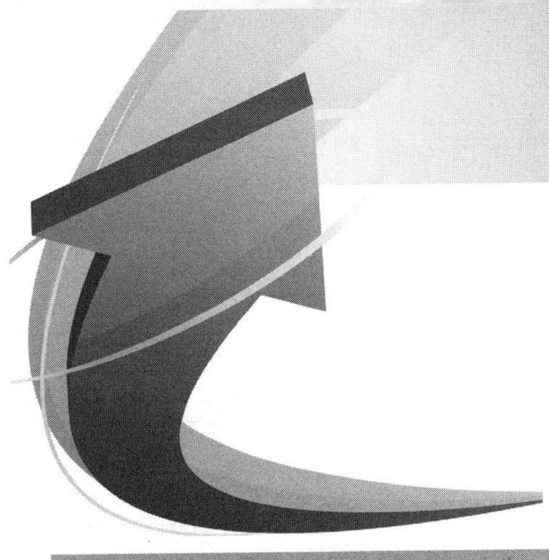

CASE 1.8
Acute Otitis Media | Level 1

Demographics

PATIENT NAME: Katie Taylor

AGE: 1 year

SEX: Female

HEIGHT: 2′4″

WEIGHT: 8.8 kg

RACE: White

ALLERGIES: NKDA

CHIEF COMPLAINT: K. T. is a 1-year-old infant brought to her pediatrician's office with complaints of a fever, irritability, and decreased oral intake.

HISTORY OF PRESENT ILLNESS: K. T. had been in her usual state of good health until the past 48 hours. Her mother states that she became irritable, is not sleeping on her usual schedule, and is refusing her usual feedings. K. T. felt warm to touch (temperature 102.3°F) to the mother this morning.

REVIEW OF SYSTEMS: Negative except as noted previously

PAST MEDICAL HISTORY: Born at term via uncomplicated standard vaginal delivery; right acute otitis media (AOM) 4 months ago (first episode); immunizations up-to-date

SOCIAL HISTORY: Lives at home with her parents and older sister (age 3 years); attends day care 5 days a week; father smokes outside; no animals in the home or outside; breastfed until 9 months of age and is now on formula and transitioning to solid foods

FAMILY HISTORY: Maternal grandmother—HTN; father—asthma; sister—asthma

Physical Examination

GEN: WDWN white female, fussy and crying

VS: BP 92/56 mm Hg, HR 124 bpm, RR 24 rpm, T 101.8°F, Wt 8.8 kg, Ht 2′4″

HEENT: Right tympanic membrane red and bulging, immobile

CHEST: Unremarkable

CV: RRR

ABD: Palpable, nontender

NEURO: WNL

EXT: WNL

Laboratory and Diagnostic Tests

WNL

Diagnosis

AOM (right ear)

Medication Record

3 MONTHS AGO

Motrin (100 mg/5 mL) 4 mL po q 8 hr prn pain/irritability

Amoxicillin (400 mg/5 mL) 1 tsp po bid × 10 days

SELF-ASSESSMENT QUESTIONS

1. Name the most common organisms that cause AOM.
2. A resident asks you about the use of TMP/SMX in AOM. How would you respond?
3. Describe the mechanism of how *Streptococcus pneumoniae* develops antimicrobial resistance to beta-lactam antimicrobials.
4. Name at least four risk factors for a higher incidence of or increase the risk of developing AOM.
5. K. T. returns to her pediatrician 3 days after the initial visit. She is still having fever and is irritable. Her mother was adherent with the antibiotic treatment. The physician feels she failed amoxicillin therapy due to a resistant organism and asks you to develop a therapeutic plan for K. T. What do you suggest?
6. What immunizations should K. T. receive at her 1-year-of-age pediatrician visit?

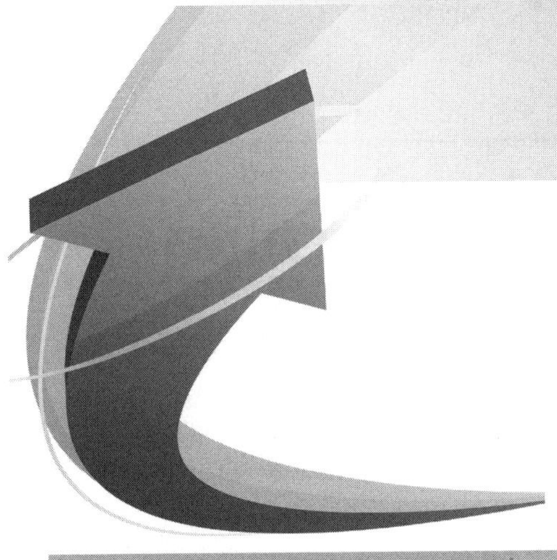

CASE 1.9
Acute Otitis Externa | Level 1

Demographics

PATIENT NAME: Lori Robertson

AGE: 17

SEX: Female

HEIGHT: 5′4″

WEIGHT: 54 kg

RACE: White

ALLERGIES: Grass and tree pollen

CHIEF COMPLAINT: L. R. is a 17-year-old female who presents to her PCP with redness and tenderness of her left ear.

HISTORY OF PRESENT ILLNESS: L. R. states that she has noticed that her left ear has been "hurting" for approximately 1 week. Over the past few days, her ear has become increasingly tender and somewhat red ("raw," as she describes it) to the point where she cannot lie on her left side or put in her earrings. She states that her ear "feels full" but denies any loss of hearing.

REVIEW OF SYSTEMS: Ear as described above; denies any headache, blurred vision, photophobia, fever, facial or neck stiffness or tenderness, or jaw/tooth pain

PAST MEDICAL HISTORY: Febrile seizures as an infant; asthma; mild facial acne; menarche at age 13

SOCIAL HISTORY: Lives with her parents and a cat in southern Texas; swims in high school and spends extended periods of time in the pool; is sexually active with a single, male partner; tobacco use—has tried tobacco but denies regular use; alcohol use—none; illicit drug use—has tried marijuana but denies regular use

FAMILY HISTORY: Parents—alive and well; mother—asthma; father—HTN

Physical Examination

GEN: Healthy-looking female in mild distress due to otalgia

VS: BP 100/70 mm Hg, HR 82 bpm, RR 20 rpm, T 37.0°C (oral), Wt 54 kg

HEENT: NC/AT, PERRLA; examination of the left external ear reveals a tender, erythematous, macerated ear canal; no obvious pus, tympanic membrane is intact; no apparent involvement of surrounding tissues; right ear normal

Neck: No stiffness; mild cervical lymphadenopathy

Lungs: CTA

Neuro: CN II-XII intact

Laboratory and Diagnostic Tests

Gram stain and microscopic examination of a swab of the external ear canal revealed gram-positive cocci in clusters. No hyphae or WBCs were seen.

Diagnosis

Acute otitis externa

Medication Record

Home Medications

Ortho-Novum 1/28, 1 tablet po daily

Claritin 10 mg po daily

Ventolin HFA 2 puffs q 4 hr prn cough or shortness of breath

Benzoyl peroxide 10% gel apply to face prn

Naproxen 220 mg po q 12 hr prn menstrual cramps

SELF-ASSESSMENT QUESTIONS

1. List risk factors and the diagnostic criteria for acute otitis externa.
2. Describe the most common organisms that cause acute otitis externa and develop a general treatment plan for L. R.
3. What if L. R.'s tympanic membrane was ruptured? Which of the following is an appropriate otic product that may be used when the tympanic membrane is perforated?
   a. Ofloxacin otic solution
   b. Antipyrine/benzocaine otic solution
   c. Ciprofloxacin/hydrocortisone otic solution
   d. Neomycin/hydrocortisone/polymyxin B otic solution
   e. Acetic acid otic solution
4. Describe techniques that a patient should be instructed to do to enhance the contact of an otic solution with the affected area.
5. The antimicrobial properties of acetic acid, which is a component of some otic preparations, are attributable to its ________.
   a. Drying properties
   b. Hypertonicity
   c. Viscosity
   d. Acidity
   e. Detergent properties
6. What are common adverse effects of antibiotics found in topical otic preparations?

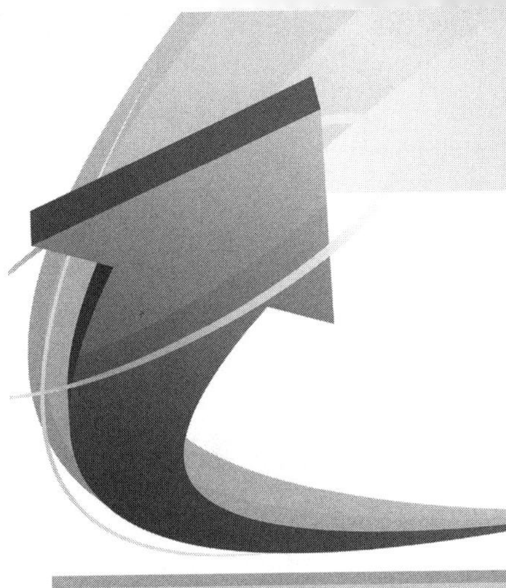

CASE 1.10
Community-Acquired Pneumonia | Level 1

Demographics

PATIENT NAME: Rebecca Thompson

AGE: 68

SEX: Female

HEIGHT: 5′6″

WEIGHT: 135 lb

RACE: White

ALLERGIES: NKDA

CHIEF COMPLAINT: R. T. is a 68-year-old white female who presented to the ED this morning at 0100 hours with a 2-day history of productive cough with fever. She also complained of shortness of breath. She decided to seek medical treatment because the chest pain and other symptoms were preventing restful sleep.

HISTORY OF PRESENT ILLNESS: Approximately 4 weeks ago, R. T. developed a UTI that was successfully treated with a 3-day course of ciprofloxacin. Following a week of being healthy, she then developed a flu-like illness of cough, malaise, and muscle aches that lasted about 10 days. While working in the yard 2 days ago, she had a sudden onset of chills, followed by fever, pleuritic chest pain, and productive cough with mucopurulent sputum. She took 400 mg of ibuprofen and an OTC cough suppressant but still had to quit working and go inside. She has remained at home resting but has not been able to sleep well since the symptoms began. She continued to take ibuprofen two to three times daily with little relief.

REVIEW OF SYSTEMS: Primary symptoms include new onset of productive cough, dyspnea, and fatigue.

PAST MEDICAL HISTORY: R. T. suffers from HTN × 7 years' duration and was recently diagnosed with diet-controlled type 2 diabetes mellitus. She has never been hospitalized and has no prior history of pneumonia.

SOCIAL HISTORY: Tobacco use—1 pack per day, 35 packs per year; alcohol use—1 to 1.5 glasses of wine per day; caffeine use—1 to 2 cups of coffee per day

Family History: Father—died at age 50 of pancreatic cancer; mother—died at age 92 of CVA; maternal grandfather—diagnosed with diabetes in his fifties; one brother living with HTN; one brother alive with no pertinent medical history; one sister deceased due to MVA

Vaccination History: Influenza vaccine last one 2 years ago; Tdap booster 5 years ago; childhood series up-to-date

Physical Examination

Gen: Well-developed female adult complaining of fatigue, malaise, and chest pain with difficulty breathing

VS: On ED admission, BP 152/88 mm Hg, HR 102 bpm, RR 26 rpm, T 39°C, Wt 61 kg

HEENT: PERRLA, throat red but without lesions

Chest: Rales heard in left lung

Neuro: Alert and oriented × 2

Laboratory and Diagnostic Tests

Sodium: 145 mEq/L

Potassium: 4.1 mEq/L

Chloride: 110 mEq/L

CO_2 Content: 25 mEq/L

BUN: 36 mg/dL

Serum Creatinine: 2.0 mg/dL

Glucose: 160 mg/dL

Hemoglobin: 14.5 g/dL

Hematocrit: 44%

Platelets: 220,000 cells/mm^3

WBC: 15,000 cells/mm^3 with 82% PMNs, 9% bands, 9% lymphocytes

CXR: Left lower lobe infiltrate

Sputum Gram Stain: Demonstrated less than 10 squamous epithelial cells and greater than 25 PMNs per low power field (LPF) with a predominance of gram-positive cocci in pairs and chains; culture is pending

O_2 Saturation on Room Air: 88%

Diagnosis

Community-acquired pneumonia

Medication Record

Home Medications

Hydrochlorothiazide 25 mg daily

Ramipril 5 mg daily

OTC ibuprofen 2 tablets prn for aches, pains, and fevers

MVI w/ minerals qam

SELF-ASSESSMENT QUESTIONS

1. What are signs and symptoms of community-acquired pneumonia, and what is the most commonly identified pathogen?
2. All of the following are indicative of an acceptable sputum specimen ***except*** ________.
   a. Greater than or equal to 10 squamous epithelial cells per LPF
   b. Greater than 25 PMNs per LPF
   c. Less than 10 squamous epithelial cells per LPF
   d. Ideally should be collected prior to initiating antibiotic therapy
   e. Sputum collection is not required to be performed in all patients based on the 2007 IDSA *Consensus Guidelines on the Management of Community-Acquired Pneumonia in Adults.*
3. R. T. was admitted to the general medical floor of the hospital with a diagnosis of community-acquired pneumonia. Develop an appropriate treatment regimen for R. T. What routine monitoring should be conducted?
4. The microbiology report for R. T.'s sputum culture indicates the pathogen is *Streptococcus pneumoniae* with high-level resistance to penicillin. Which antibiotic would be suitable to treat R. T.?
   a. Azithromycin
   b. Trimethoprim/sulfamethoxazole
   c. Linezolid
   d. Doxycycline
   e. Cefazolin

5. List risk factors for penicillin-resistant *S. pneumoniae*.
6. Which of the following would ***not*** be recommended as a preventative strategy for community-acquired pneumonia in R. T.?
   a. Smoking cessation
   b. One dose of Pneumovax® (PPSV23)
   c. Intramuscular Fluzone® high-dose (given annually)
   d. Intranasal FluMist® (given annually)
   e. Proper respiratory hygiene (including hand washing and potentially masks or tissues)

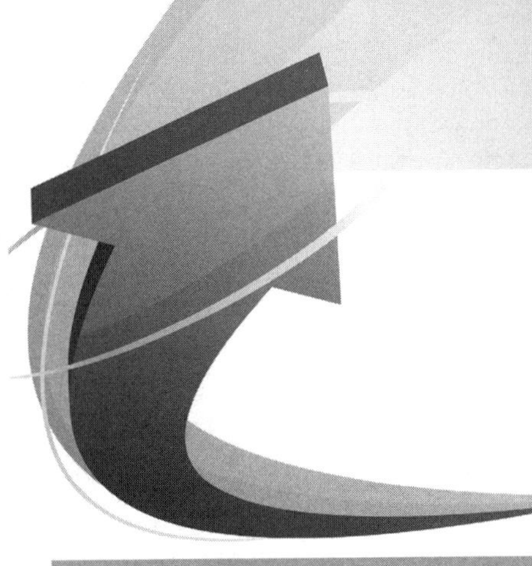

CASE 1.11
Ventilator-Associated Pneumonia | Level 2

Demographics

PATIENT NAME: Aaron Stevens

AGE: 76

SEX: Male

HEIGHT: 5′11″

WEIGHT: 177 lb

RACE: White

ALLERGIES: NKDA

CHIEF COMPLAINT: A. S. is a 76-year-old male who was admitted 13 days ago for coronary artery bypass surgery. Post CABG, the patient had a slow recovery and remained in ICU because he was unable to be extubated. Two days ago, he developed a fever and severe abdominal pain. He was subsequently taken to the operating room where a perforated duodenal ulcer was repaired. He has been stable postoperatively in the ICU. Last night, he became agitated, spiked a temperature, and had increasing oxygenation demands.

HISTORY OF PRESENT ILLNESS: Last evening, A. S. became agitated, spiked a temperature to 102.8°F, and had increasing oxygen requirements (FiO_2 increased from 40% to 80%). Two sets of blood cultures were drawn, and a sputum sample was sent for Gram stain and culture. A stat chest x-ray revealed an infiltrate at the left lower lobe.

REVIEW OF SYSTEMS: Negative except as previously noted

PAST MEDICAL HISTORY: MI 1 month ago; CABG × 5: 13 days ago; atrial fibrillation; HTN; hyperlipidemia; diabetes mellitus type 2 × 27 years; benign prostatic hypertrophy; COPD

SOCIAL HISTORY: Tobacco use—quit 35 years ago; alcohol use—occasional; marital status—married

FAMILY HISTORY: Mother—died of complications of diabetes at age 74; father—died of heart disease at age 67

Physical Examination

GEN: Elderly male, sedated, intubated

VS: BP 151/87 mm Hg, HR 93 bpm, RR 28 rpm, T 102.6°F, Wt 80.4 kg

HEENT: PERRLA, intubated

CHEST: Diminished breath sounds, rales LLL, incision pink, no drainage, healing

ABD: Incision pink, no drainage, some tenderness around incision

Laboratory and Diagnostic Tests

SODIUM: 136 mEq/L

POTASSIUM: 4.2 mEq/L

CHLORIDE: 116 mEq/L

CO_2 CONTENT: 18 mEq/L

BUN: 24 mg/dL

SERUM CREATININE: 1.2 mg/dL

GLUCOSE: 228 mg/dL

HEMOGLOBIN: 10.2 g/dL

HEMATOCRIT: 32.6%

PLATELETS: 376,000 cells/mm^3

WBC: 23,500 cells/mm^3 with 68% segs, 20% bands

CXR: Left lower lobe infiltrate

MICRO: Blood cultures negative (at 12 hr)

SPUTUM GRAM STAIN: 4+ WBC, 3+ gram-negative bacilli

Diagnosis

Ventilator-associated pneumonia

Medication Record

3/16, regular insulin sliding scale

3/16, famotidine 20 mg IVPB q 12 hr (added to TPN 3/25)

3/16, enoxaparin 40 mg SC daily (held for 2 days after abdominal surgery)

3/23, ampicillin/sulbactam (Unasyn) 3 g IVPB × 1, 1.5 g q 6 hr

3/24, midazolam 1–2 mg IV q 3 hr prn agitation

3/25, morphine sulfate 2–4 mg IV q 2 hr prn pain

3/25, TPN

3/25, enalaprilat 1.25 mg IV q 6 hr prn

4/1, warfarin 5 mg po qhs

SELF-ASSESSMENT QUESTIONS

1. Which one of the following empiric treatment regimens is most appropriate for A. S.?
   a. Ceftazidime plus gentamicin plus vancomycin
   b. Vancomycin
   c. Ceftriaxone
   d. Piperacillin/tazobactam plus gentamicin
   e. Levofloxacin plus metronidazole
2. Which one of the following statements is ***not*** a risk factor for the development of antibiotic resistance?
   a. Prior antimicrobial agent use
   b. Antimicrobial stewardship
   c. Prolonged hospitalization
   d. ICU stay
   e. Underdosage of antimicrobial agents
3. The sputum sample grows out *Pseudomonas aeruginosa*. Susceptibilities are as follows:

Drug	MIC	Breakpoint
Meropenem	0.5	≤ 2
Ceftazidime	4	≤ 8
Ciprofloxacin	2	≤ 1
Piperacillin	4	≤ 16
Gentamicin	1	≤ 4

   On the basis of the above culture and susceptibility data, which regimen is now most appropriate for A. S.?
   a. Piperacillin/tazobactam
   b. Ceftazidime plus gentamicin
   c. Meropenem plus gentamicin
   d. Ciprofloxacin plus gentamicin
   e. Ciprofloxacin
4. Two days later, you are on rounds and notice that A. S.'s serum creatinine has increased from 1.2 mg/dL to 2.4 mg/dL. Which of the following statements regarding his antimicrobial therapy is true? (He is currently receiving meropenem

2 g IVPB every 8 hours and gentamicin 160 mg IVPB every 12 hours.)

a. Change regimen to piperacillin/tazobactam plus tobramycin
b. Consider discontinuation of gentamicin
c. Recommend that the meropenem dose/interval be adjusted to 1 g every 12 hours
d. Change regimen to ciprofloxacin
e. Both b and c

5. A physician orders ceftazidime 2 g IVPB every 8 hours for a patient with an *Enterobacter* species nosocomial pneumonia. Susceptibility testing shows that the pathogen is susceptible to ceftazidime. The patient initially responds to therapy but subsequently worsens. What has potentially happened?

a. *Enterobacter* possesses an inducible beta-lactamase gene (type I beta-lactamase enzyme) that in the presence of a beta-lactam induces this enzyme.
b. Alteration in DNA gyrase is causing resistance.
c. Underdosage of the ceftazidime has induced resistance.
d. Nonadherence
e. Ceftazidime does not penetrate into the lung.

6. Which of the following oral antibiotics could be used to complete treatment of pneumonia for A. S. as an outpatient?

a. Meropenem
b. Cefuroxime
c. Amoxicillin/clavulanate
d. Ciprofloxacin
e. Moxifloxacin

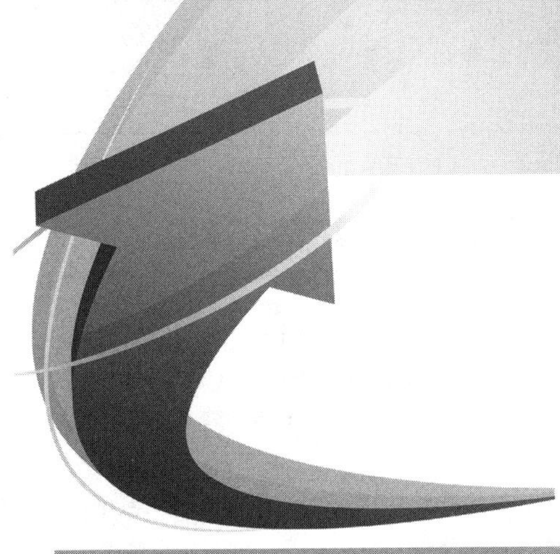

CASE 1.12
Influenza | Level 2

Demographics

Patient Name: Tina Douglas

Age: 56

Sex: Female

Height: 5′7″

Weight: 65 kg

Race: White

Allergies: Sulfa (rash)

Chief Complaint: T. D. is a 56-year-old female who presents to her physician with a 1-day history of fever, weakness, and body aches.

History of Present Illness: T. D. reports fevers to 102°F that caused her to call in sick at work today. T. D. also reports that her appetite has been poor and she "hurts all over." She has tried to increase her fluid intake but states that she just doesn't feel like eating or drinking anything. She babysat her 2-year-old grandson this weekend, and he was diagnosed with the flu yesterday. Fearing the flu, T. D. decided to report to her physician for an evaluation. On presentation to her physician, her temperature was 103°F.

Review of Systems: Negative except as noted previously

Past Medical History: T. D.'s only past medical history is HTN for the last 6 years and a history of a tonsillectomy at age 15.

Social History: Married; lives with husband; has two grown children; tobacco use—negative; alcohol use—rare social use; drug use—denied

Family History: Father—died of MI 10 years prior; mother—alive and well

Physical Examination

Gen: WDWN female in moderate distress

VS: On clinic presentation, BP 140/82 mm Hg, HR 100 bpm, RR 18 rpm, T 39.4°C, Wt 65 kg

HEENT: PERRLA, oral cavity without ulcers or lesions

Chest: Some coarse breath sounds noted

Abd: Soft, nontender

Neuro: Alert and oriented × 3

GU: Deferred

Laboratory and Diagnostic Tests

Sodium: 140 mEq/L

Potassium: 4.1 mEq/L

Chloride: 102 mEq/L

CO_2 Content: 26 mEq/L

BUN: 16 mg/dL

Serum Creatinine: 0.8 mg/dL

Glucose: 100 mg/dL

Hemoglobin: 13.1 g/dL

Hematocrit: 39.3%

Platelets: 270,000 cells/mm^3

WBC: 5,900 cells/mm^3 with 50% segs, 1% bands, 40% lymphocytes, 9% monocytes

Nasopharyngeal Swab: Positive for influenza A virus

Diagnosis

Influenza

Medication Record

Home Medications

Tylenol 500 mg po prn

Enalapril 20 mg po daily

Aspirin 325 mg po daily for CAD prevention

SELF-ASSESSMENT QUESTIONS

1. What agents are recommended by the Centers for Disease Control and Prevention (CDC) for treatment and/or prophylaxis against influenza?
2. What is the mechanism of action of the neuraminidase inhibitors?
3. Develop an appropriate treatment plan for T. D. at this time.
4. What, if any, clinical benefit is likely to be seen by starting antiviral treatment in T. D. at this time?
5. Which of the following patients would be an appropriate candidate for vaccination with a standard dose, inactivated influenza vaccine?
   a. A 3-month-old healthy infant
   b. A 45-year-old man with a history of an anaphylactic reaction to the inactivated influenza vaccine
   c. A 28-year-old pregnant woman
   d. A 15-year-old with a moderate-to-severe illness associated with fever
   e. A 68-year-old woman who developed Guillain-Barré syndrome within 6 weeks of receiving the influenza vaccine in the past
6. Which patient groups are candidates for the quadrivalent, live attenuated influenza vaccine?

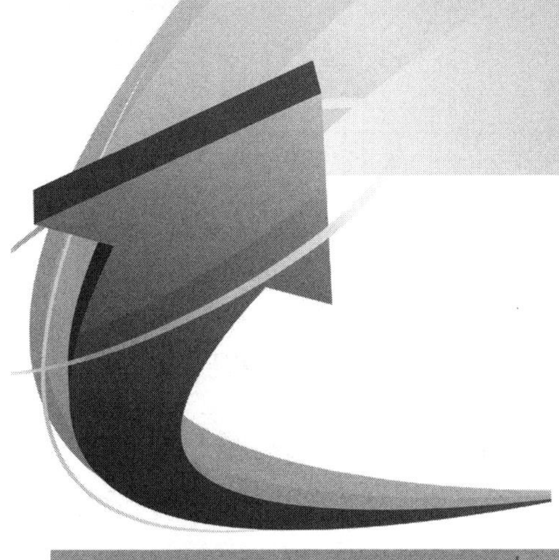

CASE 1.13
Tuberculosis | Level 3

Demographics

PATIENT NAME: Melanie Bossier

AGE: 55

SEX: Female

HEIGHT: 5′6″

WEIGHT: 155 lb

RACE: Caucasian

ALLERGIES: NKDA

CHIEF COMPLAINT: M. B. is a 55-year-old white female seen in her doctor's office yesterday afternoon complaining of weight loss and shortness of breath with exertion.

HISTORY OF PRESENT ILLNESS: M. B. notes that for the past few months she has had a low-grade temperature, has been awakened often during the night because of excessive sweating, and has had a weight loss of about 20 lb over the past 2 months. M. B.'s husband complains that during this period of time, she has also been coughing constantly. M. B. admits to occasionally coughing up blood during these coughing attacks. Upon further questioning, she mentions recently spending a 4-day vacation with her sister and family of four at their cabin near Lake Tahoe, California.

REVIEW OF SYSTEMS: Negative except as noted previously

PAST MEDICAL HISTORY: M. B. is postmenopausal and has a diagnosis of mild HTN, hypothyroidism, and gout, which are being adequately managed with her current medication regimen.

SOCIAL HISTORY: M. B. is married and has a grown daughter and five grandchildren who live with her. She is not a smoker but regularly drinks at least 1 glass of wine or beer with dinner.

FAMILY HISTORY: Noncontributory

Physical Examination

VS: T 99.8°F, HR 84 bpm, RR 24 rpm, BP 135/72 mm Hg

SKIN/EXT: No rash, cyanosis, clubbing, or edema

NECK: Supple, no lymphadenopathy

LUNGS: Bibasilar rales and apical "crackles" on deep inspiration

NEURO: Alert and oriented × 3

Laboratory and Diagnostic Tests

WBC: 9,800 cells/mm^3

HEMOGLOBIN: 12 g/dL

HEMATOCRIT: 38%

SERUM CREATININE: 1.3 mg/dL

SERUM BICARBONATE: 26 mEq/L

GLUCOSE: 142 mg/dL (nonfasting)

T_4 (FREE): 1.5 ng/dL

TSH: 1.6 milli-international units/L

AST: 45 international units/L

ALT: 30 international units/L

CXR: Right lower lobe infiltrate with bilateral hilar and right paratracheal adenopathy; evidence of old cavitary lesions in both apices

Diagnosis

Tuberculosis

Medication Record

Premarin (conjugated estrogen) 1.25 mg daily

Amlodipine 10 mg daily

Levothyroxine 0.15 mg daily

Allopurinol 300 mg daily

SELF-ASSESSMENT QUESTIONS

1. On the basis of the information provided, tuberculin screening skin tests (PPD) should be given to which family members?
2. The patient's husband has a positive reaction within 48 hours of administration of a PPD skin test. What is considered a positive reaction of a PPD skin test?
3. Which one of the following statements is ***false*** regarding the QuantiFERON-TB Gold In-Tube test (QFT-GIT)?
   a. It may be used to diagnose both latent and active TB infections.
   b. QFT-GIT should be used in place of a PPD skin test, but ***not*** in addition to a PPD skin test.
   c. A prior BCG (Bacillus Calmette–Guérin) vaccination does ***not*** cause a false-positive result.
   d. The patient must return to clinic within 48 to 72 hours to assess the reaction.
   e. QFT-GIT is not preferred over a PPD in children less than 5 years of age.
4. What is an initial appropriate treatment recommendation for M. B.'s pulmonary TB disease? In addition to the specific anti-TB regimen selected, what other therapy should be considered for M. B. at this time?
5. M. B.'s liver function tests increase to two times the original concentrations after 1 month of therapy with isoniazid, rifampin, pyrazinamide, and ethambutol. M. B. does not have any complaints regarding her drug therapy, other than having to take so many drugs in a single day. Which of the following should ***not*** be a recommended change to her drug therapy?
   a. Decrease the dose of isoniazid to half the starting dose; discontinue the rifampin.
   b. Interview the patient monthly for symptoms of hepatotoxicity.
   c. Inform the patient of symptoms of hepatotoxicity and tell her to report these to her doctor if they occur.
   d. Maintain the original doses of isoniazid, rifampin, and pyrazinamide.
   e. Monitor liver function tests for the entire course of therapy.
6. One of M. B.'s grandchildren has a positive reaction to the PPD skin test. What therapy, if any, should be initiated in this 6-year-old male who is otherwise healthy and without clinical evidence of TB?

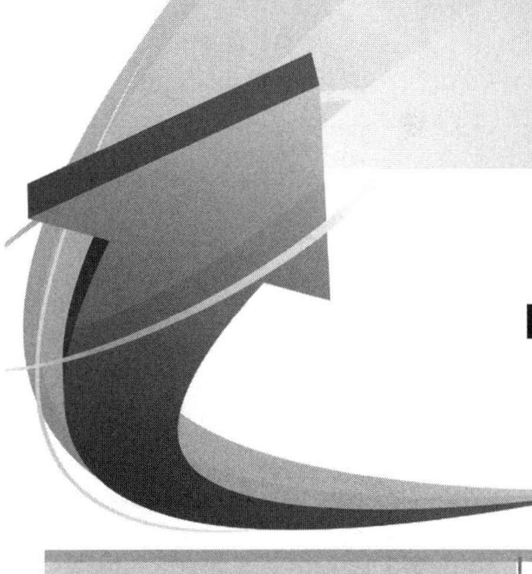

CASE 1.14
Healthcare-Associated Pneumonia | Level 3

Demographics

PATIENT NAME: Victor Thompson

AGE: 59

SEX: Male

HEIGHT: 5′5″

WEIGHT: 160 lb

RACE: White

ALLERGIES: NKDA

CHIEF COMPLAINT: V. T. is a 59-year-old male who presented to the ED by EMS after an apparent seizure he had at his group home around 2 p.m. today.

HISTORY OF PRESENT ILLNESS: Currently, the patient is very drowsy and unable to answer questions consistently. He is oriented only to self and place. No caregivers are in attendance, and he is a poor historian. He reports pain in his chest on the right side. The patient was recently seen in the ED 3 days ago for a sore throat, fever, and rhinorrhea. He was presumed to have acute pharyngitis and was administered penicillin G benzathine 1.2 million units IM × 1.

REVIEW OF SYSTEMS: Unable to obtain

PAST MEDICAL HISTORY: HTN, COPD, bipolar disorder

SOCIAL HISTORY: Tobacco use—quit 2 years ago, smoked 2 packs per day for 35 years; denies alcohol or illicit drug use; marital status—single; has lived in a group home the past 8 years

FAMILY HISTORY: Unknown

VACCINE HISTORY: Td 6 years ago; influenza 4 years ago; childhood series up-to-date

Physical Examination

GEN: Middle-aged male, very drowsy, oriented to self and place

VS: BP 117/62 mm Hg, HR 111 bpm, RR 18 rpm, T 98.3°F, Wt 160 lb

HEENT: PERRLA but sluggish, face flushed not compliant with neuro exam so cannot fully assess EOM; will not open mouth for evaluation

Chest: Tachycardia with no m/r/g appreciated, bilateral course inspiratory crackles and rhonchi, crackles locally increased to right lower lobe

Abd: Soft, nontender, obese, BS normal

Ext: 2+ pulses, no CCE

Laboratory and Diagnostic Tests

Sodium: 138 mEq/L

Potassium: 3.9 mEq/L

Chloride: 93 mEq/L

CO_2 Content: 30 mEq/L

BUN: 21 mg/dL

Serum Creatinine: 1.67 mg/dL

Glucose: 132 mg/dL

Calcium: 9.8 mg/dL

Hemoglobin: 13.4 g/dL

Hematocrit: 41.6%

Platelets: 298,000 cells/mm^3

WBC: 16,200 cells/mm^3 with 68% segs, 20% bands

CXR: Right lower lobe infiltrate, not seen on CXR 72 hours prior

ECG: Sinus tachycardia with PVCs, QTc 527

pH: 7.269, HCO_3 35.8, pCO_2 78, pO_2 45

Diagnosis

Healthcare-associated pneumonia (HCAP)

Medication Record

Home Medications

Albuterol 2 puffs q 6 hr prn wheezing or SOB

Clonidine 0.2 mg po bid

Fluoxetine 20 mg po daily

Olanzapine 15 mg ODT qhs

Hydrocodone/homatropine 1 tsp po qid prn cough

Inpatient Medications

Piperacillin/tazobactam 3.375 g IVPB × 1

Vancomycin 20 mg/kg IVPB × 1

SELF-ASSESSMENT QUESTIONS

1. The medical resident needs to initiate therapy for V. T. and asks if he should administer ceftriaxone alone or a combination of levofloxacin and vancomycin. What is the best response to the resident?
2. Which antibiotics potentially used for HCAP have postantibiotic effects?
3. What if you had a patient with pneumonia and *Acinetobacter* spp. was the causative pathogen, what antibiotics are the most active against this species?
4. What should the clinician do if the patient is not responding to initial therapy?
5. In evaluating his vaccine record, does V. T. need any immunizations at this time or in the future?
6. If V. T. had a history of experiencing shortness of breath with amoxicillin use, what medication would have been an appropriate treatment for the presumed acute pharyngitis?

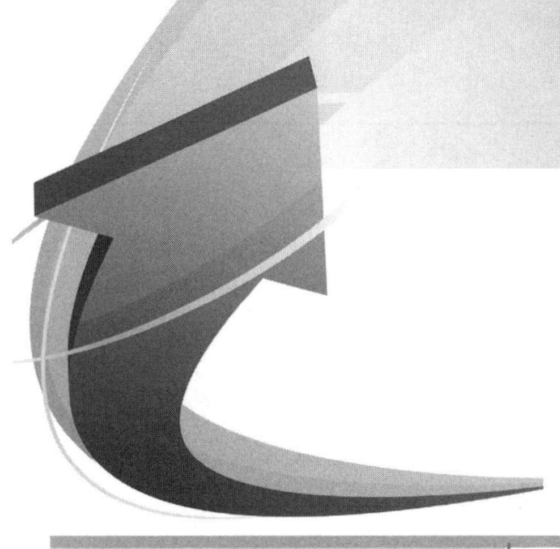

CASE 1.15
Neonatal Sepsis | Level 1

Demographics

PATIENT NAME: Baby Girl Smith

AGE: 0

SEX: Female

HEIGHT: 43.2 cm

WEIGHT: 3 lb 14 oz

RACE: Caucasian

ALLERGIES: NKDA

CHIEF COMPLAINT: Baby Girl Smith is a 31-week-old premature infant admitted to the neonatal ICU immediately after birth to rule out the possibility of sepsis.

HISTORY OF PRESENT ILLNESS: Baby Girl Smith was born by vaginal delivery at 31 weeks gestation to a 29-year-old mother (gravida 4, para 3, spontaneous Ab 1) at 12:45 p.m. today. APGAR scores were 6 and 8 at 1 and 5 minutes, respectively. Cord pH was 7.32.

REVIEW OF SYSTEMS: Negative except as previously noted

PAST MEDICAL HISTORY: Maternal history positive for rupture of membranes × 20 hours, pregnancy-induced HTN (beginning 3 weeks ago), and group B *Streptococcus* (GBS) positive; medication use during pregnancy: prenatal vitamins, Zantac, and Tylenol

MATERNAL SCREEN: GBS positive (no treatment); RPR negative; HIV negative; HBV negative; HSV negative; chlamydia negative; rubella immune

SOCIAL HISTORY: None

FAMILY HISTORY: Will live with mother, father, two sisters (ages 8 and 4), and one brother (age 2) at home; maternal grandmother—HTN; sister (age 8)—asthma

Physical Examination

GEN: Mottled color, active

VS: T 98.4°F, HR 137 bpm, RR 42 rpm, BP 43/32 mm Hg, O_2 sat 97% RA, Ht 43.2 cm, head circumference 30 cm

HEENT: Anterior fontanelle present, no cleft palate or lip

Chest: Bilateral breath sounds

CV: RRR, no murmur

Abd: Soft, NTND, positive BS

GU: Normal female genitalia, patent anus

Neuro: Good tone

Ext: 20 digits, cap refill 4 sec

Laboratory and Diagnostic Tests

Sodium: 139 mEq/L

Potassium: 5.2 mEq/L

Chloride: 108 mEq/L

CO_2 Content: 25 mEq/L

BUN: 14 mg/dL

Serum Creatinine: 0.8 mg/dL

Glucose: 60 mg/dL

Calcium: 7.2 mg/dL

Protein: 4.2 g/dL

Albumin: 2.6 g/dL

Total Bilirubin: 4.0 mg/dL

ALP: 118 units/L

AST: 50 units/L

ALT: 13 units/L

WBC: 9,800 cells/mm^3 with 52% segs, 5% bands, 38% lymphocytes, and 5% monocytes

Hemoglobin: 15.7 g/dL

Hematocrit: 46.3%

Platelets: 319,000 cells/mm^3

Blood Cultures: Pending

CSF Cultures: Pending

Diagnosis

Suspected sepsis

Medication Record

Ampicillin 176 mg IV q 12 hr

Gentamicin 7 mg IV q 48 hr

D10W at 6 mL/hr

SELF-ASSESSMENT QUESTIONS

1. What organisms are common causes of early-onset sepsis in a neonate? What organisms are common causes of late-onset sepsis in a neonate? What are the transmission methods of the organisms for early-onset and late-onset sepsis?
2. What are risk factors for early-onset sepsis and late-onset sepsis in a neonate?
3. Describe the mechanism of actions of gentamicin and ampicillin. Why are these antibiotics recommended for empiric use in early-onset sepsis?
4. Gentamicin serum levels return for Baby Girl Smith. The trough is 0.9 mcg/mL, and the peak is 7.8 mcg/mL. Levels were all drawn appropriately. How would you adjust her current dose?
5. At what time frame can discontinuing antibiotics in Baby Girl Smith be considered if she shows no signs of illness, feeds well, and cultures are negative?
6. Baby Girl Smith's blood and CSF cultures return positive for group B *Streptococcus.* What alterations do you recommend for antibiotic treatment and duration of therapy, if any?

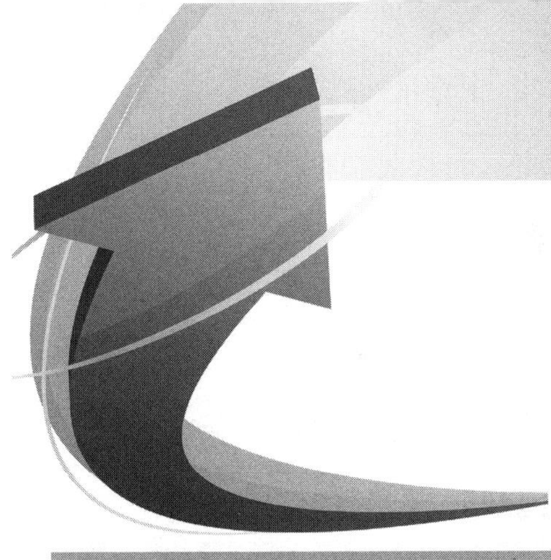

CASE 1.16
Infective Endocarditis—Viridans Group Streptococci | Level 1

Demographics

PATIENT NAME: Robert Rodriguez

AGE: 57

SEX: Male

HEIGHT: 5′7″

WEIGHT: 78 kg

RACE: Hispanic American

ALLERGIES: NKDA

CHIEF COMPLAINT: R. R. is a 57-year-old Hispanic male who was admitted to the hospital with general weakness, fever with night sweats, and dyspnea. R. R. states he feels weak and has no appetite. His daughter states her father usually is a big eater, and for the past 2 days he has not eaten and has complained of being too warm and having occasional chills.

HISTORY OF PRESENT ILLNESS: R. R. had a tooth extracted by his dentist 1 week ago, and over the past 3 to 4 days has been experiencing shortness of breath when completing activities of daily living. His activity has decreased substantially, and he has been sitting in his chair most of the day. He stated he was chilled and sweating last night. This morning, his daughter felt his forehead and he felt warm, so she gave him two acetaminophen tablets.

REVIEW OF SYSTEMS: Unremarkable

PAST MEDICAL HISTORY: R. R. has a history of mitral valve prolapse with regurgitation approximately 3 years ago. He was admitted about 11 months ago for an infective endocarditis caused by viridans group streptococci. He spent 2 weeks in the hospital, followed by 2 weeks of home healthcare. The remainder of his history is unremarkable except for HTN.

SOCIAL HISTORY: Tobacco use—none; alcohol use—none; caffeine use—1 to 2 cups of coffee in the morning; drug abuse—none

FAMILY HISTORY: Mother—died of MI at age 66; father—died of complications of surgery at age 58

Physical Examination

GEN: Pale, WD, NAD except for general weakness

VS: BP 138/95 mm Hg, HR 90 bpm, RR 28 rpm, T 38.7°C, Wt 78 kg

HEENT: Unremarkable

CHEST: Heart murmur

NEURO: Alert and oriented × 3

Laboratory and Diagnostic Tests

SODIUM: 145 mEq/L

POTASSIUM: 3.8 mEq/L

FBG: 79 mg/dL

WBC: 14,000 cells/mm^3

RBC: 4.6 cells/mm^3

HEMOGLOBIN: 13.1 g/dL

HEMATOCRIT: 42%

RETICULOCYTE COUNT: 0.5%

TIBC: 223 mg/dL

FE: 49 g/dL

BLOOD CULTURES: Microbiology reports five of six BACTEC cultures are positive for viridans group streptococci, highly susceptible to penicillin

TEE: 1.4-cm mobile vegetation on mitral valve

Diagnosis

Infective endocarditis, streptococci

Medication Record

PRIOR TO ADMISSION

Hydrochlorothiazide 25 mg po daily

Tylenol 650 mg prn

SELF-ASSESSMENT QUESTIONS

1. Which of the symptoms exhibited by R. R. would be included as a Duke criteria contributing to the diagnosis of infective endocarditis?
2. Prior to receiving microbiology blood culture results, which pathogens would you consider when selecting empiric treatment options for this patient with suspected infective endocarditis?
3. What would be the best choice for empiric treatment of the two most likely pathogens for infective endocarditis in this patient? What treatment duration is warranted?
4. What if the MIC of the viridans group streptococci was greater than 0.5 mcg/mL, resulting in a penicillin-resistant strain?
5. What would be the best antibiotic prophylaxis recommendation for a patient with a history of infective endocarditis undergoing an invasive dental procedure?
6. If the physician believes this patient experienced a penicillin-induced, nonanaphylactoid-type allergic reaction during the patient's last admission, which antibiotic would you recommend for treatment at this admission?

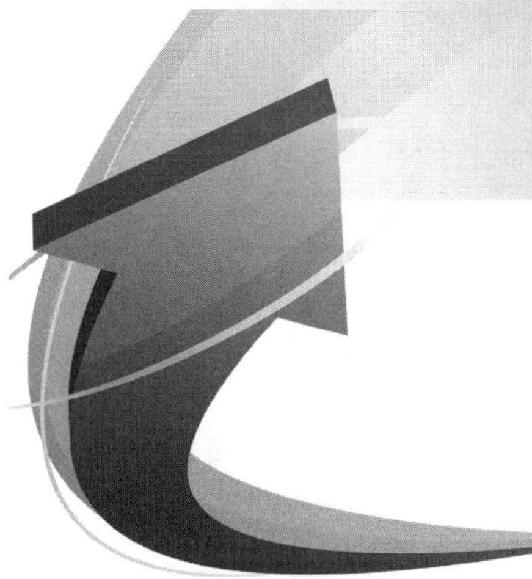

CASE 1.17
Catheter-Related Bloodstream Infection—Antibiotic Resistance | Level 2

Demographics

PATIENT NAME: Marko Ramius

AGE: 30

SEX: Male

HEIGHT: 5′10″

WEIGHT: 102 kg

RACE: Caucasian

ALLERGIES: NKDA

CHIEF COMPLAINT: M. R. was found to be diaphoretic and slightly confused by the evening staff nurse at White Oak Rehabilitation Hospital.

HISTORY OF PRESENT ILLNESS: The onset of symptoms was within the previous 8 hours; however, M. R. reported feeling "under the weather" for the past few days.

REVIEW OF SYSTEMS: Fever present; (+) anxiety; bilateral lower extremity paralysis

PAST MEDICAL HISTORY: C-6 spinal fracture secondary to motor vehicle accident 2 years ago; partial colectomy 2 years ago; hospitalized for community-acquired pneumonia 2 weeks ago; hospitalized for UTI 4 weeks ago

SOCIAL HISTORY: Not married, no children

FAMILY HISTORY: Mother, father, and two older siblings alive and well

Physical Examination

GEN: Well-nourished, ill-appearing adult male

VS: BP 90/60 mm Hg, HR 110 bpm, RR 16 rpm, T 38.5°C, Wt 102 kg, Ht 5′10″

SKIN: Subclavian catheter site is erythematous and warm to touch; multiple scars on abdomen and neck from injuries and surgery

CHEST: CTAB with no wheezes or crackles

CV: Tachycardic with no m/r/g appreciated

Abd: Soft, NTND, normoactive bowel sounds

MS/Ext: Motor and sensory activity is absent in the lower extremities and diminished in upper extremities

Neuro: A&O × 3

Laboratory and Diagnostic Tests

Sodium: 142 mEq/L

Potassium: 4.1 mEq/L

Chloride: 109 mEq/L

CO_2 Content: 21 mEq/L

BUN: 5 mg/dL

Serum Creatinine: 0.3 mg/dL

Glucose: 90 mg/dL

Gram Stain: Gram-positive cocci in clusters

Blood Cultures: (in ED) positive 2 out of 2 for *Staphylococcus aureus*; susceptibilities pending

Nasal Swab: MRSA positive

Diagnosis

Catheter-related bloodstream infection

Medication Record

Piperacillin/tazobactam 4.5 g IV q 6 hr

Vancomycin 1 g IV q 12 hr

Pantoprazole 40 mg IV q 24 hr

Heparin 5,000 units SC q 12 hr

Baclofen 10 mg po tid

Docusate sodium 100 mg po bid

Morphine 2 mg IV q 2 hr prn pain

Senna 8.6 mg 1 tablet po qpm prn constipation

Bisacodyl suppository 10 mg pr qpm prn constipation

SELF-ASSESSMENT QUESTIONS

1. Suppose the organism isolated in M. R.'s blood cultures returned as susceptible to oxacillin but resistant to penicillin G. Which of the following would be the most likely mechanism of resistance?
   a. Production of penicillinase
   b. Production of a penicillin efflux pump
   c. Alteration of penicillin-binding protein 2a
   d. Alteration of DNA gyrase
   e. Loss of a porin channel in the outer membrane
2. Suppose the organism isolated in M. R.'s blood cultures returned as susceptible to vancomycin but resistant to oxacillin. Which of the following would be the most likely mechanism of resistance?
   a. Change from D-ala-D-ala to D-ala-D-lactate
   b. Alteration of penicillin-binding protein 2a
   c. Production of an extended-spectrum beta-lactamase
   d. Efflux of beta-lactam antibiotics
   e. Alteration of the 50S ribosomal subunit
3. Suppose the organism isolated in M. R.'s blood cultures returned as MSSA susceptible to clindamycin and quinupristin/dalfopristin but resistant to erythromycin. Which of the following would be the most likely mechanism of resistance?
   a. Change from D-ala-D-ala to D-ala-D-lactate
   b. Alteration of penicillin-binding protein 2a
   c. Production of an extended-spectrum beta-lactamase
   d. Efflux of macrolide antibiotics
   e. Alteration of the 50S ribosomal subunit
4. Suppose the organism isolated in M. R.'s blood cultures returned with a susceptibility profile suggesting a community-associated MRSA strain. Which antibiotic would be most appropriate for M. R. and at what dosing regimen? Does the catheter need to be removed?

5. The third-year medical student asks you if antibiotic lock therapy could be used to treat this patient. How do you respond?
6. Which of the following strategies would be most effective for preventing future catheter-related bloodstream infections in M. R.?
   a. Changing the catheter site to the internal jugular vein
   b. Administering IV vancomycin for prophylaxis
   c. Flushing the catheter daily with heparin
   d. Using an inline filter when infusing drugs
   e. Using aseptic technique when inserting a new catheter

CASE 1.18
Infective Endocarditis—*Staphylococcus* | Level 2

Demographics

PATIENT NAME: Lane Peterson

AGE: 37

SEX: Male

HEIGHT: 5′10″

WEIGHT: 67 kg

RACE: Caucasian

ALLERGIES: NKDA

CHIEF COMPLAINT: General weakness, fever with night sweats, and dyspnea on exertion. L. P. states he has not felt like himself for the past few days with general aches and pains. Today he felt like he was running a fever and decided to come to the ED on his own.

HISTORY OF PRESENT ILLNESS: L. P. is a homeless person and known IV drug abuser. He has felt weak for the past 3 days with general aches and pains when he gets up to walk around. L. P. has experienced night sweats for the past 2 nights. L. P. feels chilled; however, this is not uncommon for him during the winter season. L. P. states he has not eaten in the past 2 days. Today, he felt warmer and thought he might have an infection because his arm has been red and swollen for a few days.

REVIEW OF SYSTEMS: Coughing, diaphoretic, multiple track marks on right antecubital area

PAST MEDICAL HISTORY: Admission 3 years ago for ORIF of left tibial fracture. During that admission, a urine drug screen was positive for heroin and cocaine. There were two ED visits in the past 12 months for contusions, lacerations, and abrasions on his face, shoulder, and knee requiring debridement and sutures.

SOCIAL HISTORY: Tobacco use—2 packs per day; alcohol use—pint of whisky per day; drug use—known IVDA, last use was 5 days ago

FAMILY HISTORY: Mother and father—died in an MVA at ages 61 and 62, respectively; no brothers or sisters

Physical Examination

GEN: Pale, malnourished thin male, IV tracks on arms and legs, body lice

VS: On admission to the ED, BP 138/80 mm Hg, HR 97 bpm, RR 27 rpm, T 39.3°C, Wt 67 kg

HEENT: Unremarkable

CHEST: Diastolic heart murmur

NEURO: Slow to respond and oriented × 2

Laboratory and Diagnostic Tests

SODIUM: 139 mEq/L

POTASSIUM: 3.8 mEq/L

SERUM CREATININE: 1.0 mg/dL

FBG: 76 mg/dL

WBC: 2,600 cells/mm^3

POLYS: 80%

BANDS: 9%

HEMOGLOBIN: 14 g/dL

HEMATOCRIT: 40%

BLOOD CULTURES: Three sets of two cultures drawn by venipuncture were collected over a 1-hour period. Preliminary culture shows gram-positive cocci in clusters in four of six cultures; final organism identification and sensitivities are pending.

CHEST X-RAY: Results pending

ECHOCARDIOGRAPHY: TTE ordered

Diagnosis

Infective endocarditis

Medication Record

None available

SELF-ASSESSMENT QUESTIONS

1. What are risk factors for infective endocarditis from *Streptococcus*, *Staphylococcus*, and *Enterococcus* organisms?
2. Compare and contrast transesophageal echocardiogram (TEE) to transthoracic echocardiogram (TTE) for the evaluation of infective endocarditis.
3. If blood cultures identify methicillin-sensitive *Staphylococcus* in a patient with known or suspected infective endocarditis, what antibiotic therapy should be initiated?
4. What is the recommended gentamicin dose for endocarditis caused by methicillin-sensitive *Staphylococcus aureus* (MSSA) in a patient with normal renal function? What are the target gentamicin peak and trough concentrations in the treatment of gram-positive cocci endocarditis?
5. The most recent microbiology sensitivity report noted growth of methicillin-resistant *Staphylococcus aureus* (MRSA), and the patient continues to have a low-grade fever. What drug regimen would you recommend to the prescribing physician?
6. For which of the following patient factors would infective endocarditis prophylaxis be reasonable for a patient undergoing an invasive dental procedure where bleeding from gingival tissue is expected to occur?
   a. Heart failure
   b. Mitral valve prolapse without valve dysfunction
   c. Atrial septal defect
   d. Cardiac pacemaker
   e. Previous endocarditis

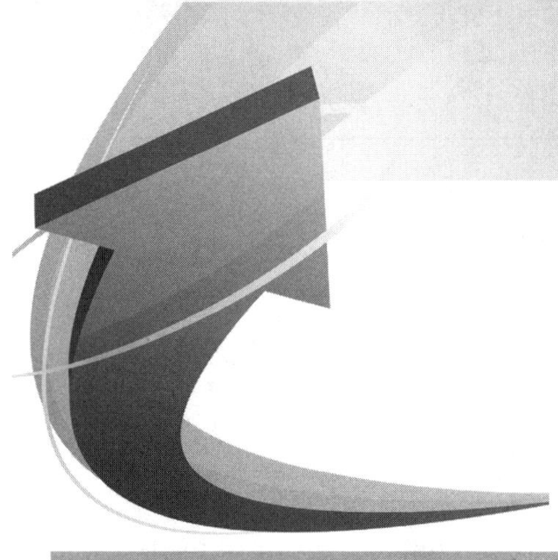

CASE 1.19
Bacteremia, Gram Positive | Level 2

Demographics

PATIENT NAME: Michelle Clemens

AGE: 67

SEX: Female

HEIGHT: 5′4″

WEIGHT: 161 lb

RACE: African American

ALLERGIES: sulfa (rash-macular and papular eruption)

CHIEF COMPLAINT: M. C. is a 67-year-old female hospitalized 1 week ago for coronary bypass surgery after suffering an acute MI. She had an uneventful postoperative period and is currently in the step-down unit, where you are the clinical pharmacist.

HISTORY OF PRESENT ILLNESS: This morning, M. C. spiked a temperature of 102.6°F. The nurse also noticed an area of erythema and swelling around her central line during a routine dressing change. The central line was replaced, and two sets of blood cultures were drawn. One specimen of each set was obtained via the central line, and one specimen was taken from a peripheral venipuncture. These specimens were sent for Gram stain, culture, and sensitivity.

REVIEW OF SYSTEMS: A 67-year-old, African-American female post-operative for triple-vessel bypass presents this morning with fever and erythema, swelling, and tenderness at the site of a central line.

PAST MEDICAL HISTORY: M. C. has a 20-year history of HTN that has been moderately controlled with various agents. In the last 6 months, M. C. had been complaining of increased shortness of breath and mild angina. She had a cholecystectomy at age 25 and had two children via normal vaginal delivery at age 24 and 28.

SOCIAL HISTORY: Tobacco use—quit 25 years ago; alcohol use—none; marital status—married

FAMILY HISTORY: Father—died of heart disease at age 63; mother—died of breast cancer at age 69

Physical Examination

VS: This morning, BP 144/88 mm Hg, HR 80 bpm, RR 25 rpm, T 102.6°F, Wt 161 lb; area around central venous IV site is erythematous and indurated

Laboratory and Diagnostic Tests

Sodium: 142 mEq/L

Potassium: 4.2 mEq/L

Chloride: 110 mEq/L

CO_2 Content: 30 mEq/L

BUN: 15 mg/dL

Serum Creatinine: 1.2 mg/dL

Glucose: 141 mg/dL

AST: 15 international units/L

ALT: 19 international units/L

Hemoglobin: 12.1 g/dL

Hematocrit: 35%

Platelets: 250,000 cells/mm^3

WBC: 21,000 cells/mm^3 with 60% PMNs, 6% bands

ECG: NSR

CXR: Patchy infiltrates consistent with HF

Micro: Gram stain—gram-positive cocci in clusters, in four of four culture specimens

Diagnosis

Bacteremia, gram positive

Medication Record

Home Medications

Metoprolol 100 mg 1 tablet po bid

Losartan 50 mg 1 tablet po daily

Atorvastatin 10 mg 1 tablet po daily

MVI 1 tablet po daily

Vitamin E 400 international units 1 capsule po daily

Inpatient Medication Record

Cefazolin 1 g IVPB preop × 1

Cefazolin 1 g IVPB q 8 hr (D/C'd)

Vancomycin 1 g IV q12 hr

Metoprolol 100 mg po bid

Losartan 50 mg po daily

Atorvastatin 10 mg po daily

Morphine 1–2 mg IV q 4 hr prn severe pain

APAP 325/oxycodone 5 mg po q 4 hr prn moderate pain

SELF-ASSESSMENT QUESTIONS

1. An M4 medical student asks you about guidelines for preventing central catheter-related infections. Which of the following would be an appropriate recommendation?
   a. Promptly remove any intravascular catheter that is no longer essential.
   b. Change tunneled catheter site dressings every 2 days until the site has healed.
   c. Give a dose of prophylactic antibiotics 1 hour before catheter insertion.
   d. Replace the central venous catheter every 2 weeks.
   e. Use a vancomycin antibiotic lock solution for all idle central catheter ports.
2. What antimicrobial agents and duration should be used first line for bacteremia?
3. The attending physician started M. C. on vancomycin therapy. When monitoring vancomycin serum concentrations, what is the recommended trough level range for the treatment of bacteremia?
4. You receive a call from M. C.'s nurse stating that M. C. became slightly hypotensive (110/60 mm Hg) and developed a rash on her trunk and arms when receiving her first dose of vancomycin. What actions do you recommend?
5. By day 7 of therapy with vancomycin, M. C. is clinically stable, but a recent chemistry panel shows an increase in her serum creatinine to 1.9 mg/dL. Assuming that the bacteria was found to be methicillin-resistant *Staphylococcus aureus* (MRSA) and the patient was going to be continued on IV vancomycin, how would you empirically dose the drug in this patient?

6. After 10 days on IV vancomycin, the medical fellow wants to convert this patient to oral vancomycin. He wants to know whether an oral formulation of vancomycin is available and what the most appropriate dose is for this patient. What is the best response?

7. If the bacteria causing the patient's infection are determined to be methicillin-sensitive *Staphylococcus aureus* (MSSA), what antibiotic would be the optimal choice for treatment?

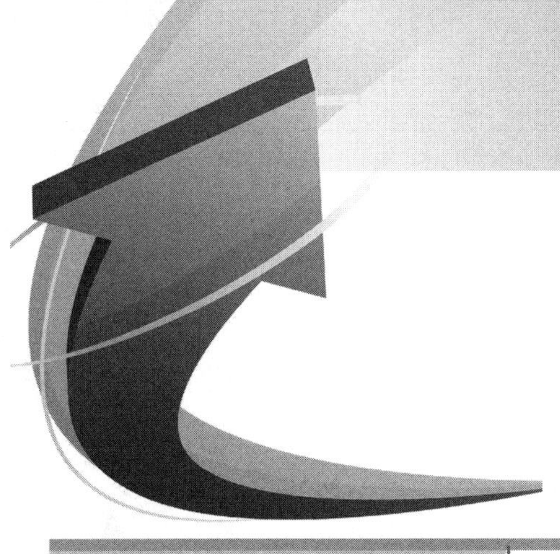

CASE 1.20
Bacteremia, Gram Negative | Level 3

Demographics

PATIENT NAME: Micha Morris

AGE: 32

SEX: Male

HEIGHT: 6′4″

WEIGHT: 210 lb

RACE: White

ALLERGIES: Sulfa (erythema multiforme)

CHIEF COMPLAINT: M. M. is a 32-year-old male who was admitted to the hospital 4 days ago as the result of a motorcycle accident. He presented with a closed head injury, multiple fractures involving both upper and lower extremities, and internal injuries requiring emergent surgery. He was transferred to the surgical ICU postoperatively, where he has remained in critical but stable condition. Today his temperature spiked to 104.1°F.

HISTORY OF PRESENT ILLNESS: M. M. was involved in a motorcycle versus automobile accident 4 days ago. He presented with a closed head injury; fractures of the left femur, left tibia, and left humerus; and internal bleeding for which he underwent an emergency exploratory laparotomy. There were several lacerations on his liver that were repaired, and his spleen was removed. He was transferred to the surgical ICU postoperatively, where he remained intubated, requiring dopamine for the first 24 hours to maintain his blood pressure. Since that time, he has been in critical but stable condition, not requiring any pressors for blood pressure support. This morning, his temperature spiked to 104°F, and his blood pressure dropped to 90/65 mm Hg.

REVIEW OF SYSTEMS: Negative except as noted previously

PAST MEDICAL HISTORY: Depression; HTN

SOCIAL HISTORY: Married with a 6-year-old son; tobacco—none; alcohol use—4 drinks per week

FAMILY HISTORY: Both parents alive and in good health; no siblings

Physical Examination

GEN: Flushed, diaphoretic young male, intubated, in moderate distress

VS: BP 90/65 mm Hg, HR 120 bpm, RR 28 rpm, T 104.1°F, Wt 210 lb

HEENT: PERRLA, intubated

CHEST: Breath sounds bilaterally, some dullness on the right side

Laboratory and Diagnostic Test

SODIUM: 138 mEq/L

POTASSIUM: 3.9 mEq/L

CHLORIDE: 114 mEq/L

CO_2 CONTENT: 28 mEq/L

BUN: 20 mg/dL

SERUM CREATININE: 1.5 mg/dL

GLUCOSE: 153 mg/dL

HEMOGLOBIN: 14.4 g/dL

HEMATOCRIT: 37%

PLATELETS: 278,000 cells/mm^3

WBC: 25,000 cells/mm^3 with 50% PMNs, 11% bands

CXR: Some consolidation noted on right side

MICRO: Gram-negative rods from tracheal aspirate and gram-negative rods from one of two blood cultures

NOTE: ICU has experienced a significant increase in ESBL+ GNB isolates, including *Klebsiella*, *E. coli*, *Enterobacter*, and *Pseudomonas*.

Diagnosis

Bacteremia, gram-negative

Medication Record

HOME MEDICATIONS

Multivitamin daily

Lisinopril 20 mg po daily

Venlafaxine extended-release 75 mg po daily

Acetaminophen 325 mg, 2 tablets once or twice a week for headache

INPATIENT RECORD

4/4, cefoxitin 1 g IVPB q 6 hr

4/4, ranitidine 50 mg IVPB q 8 hr

4/4, dopamine drip IV

4/4, vecuronium drip IV

4/4, midazolam drip IV

4/4, hydromorphone 2 mg IVP q 4 hr prn

4/5, continuous TPN

SELF-ASSESSMENT QUESTIONS

1. Considering M. M.'s condition on admission and clinical course during this hospitalization, what organisms would be considered a likely potential cause of his infection when selecting empiric antimicrobial therapy?
2. After reviewing the microbiology report revealing gram-negative bacteria from two sources, what would be an appropriate empiric therapy recommendation for this patient?
3. Because the patient has had a splenectomy, which vaccine-preventable disease is he at a higher risk for contracting?
4. What would be an appropriate dose of once-daily gentamicin for this patient?
5. An M4 medical student is on trauma rotations this month, and she asks what the rationale is for dosing aminoglycosides once daily in patients that can tolerate it. You respond with a brief discussion about the pharmacodynamics of aminoglycosides. Which pharmacodynamic parameter best describes the rationale for dosing aminoglycosides once daily?
6. One of M. M.'s blood cultures is positive for *Candida glabrata*, and the on-call resident asks you for an antifungal recommendation to treat this candidemia. Which of the following should you recommend?
   a. Amphotericin B deoxycholate 3 mg/kg IV daily
   b. Fluconazole 400-mg IV loading dose, then 200 mg IV daily
   c. Terbinafine 250 mg IV daily
   d. Caspofungin 70-mg IV loading dose, then 50 mg IV daily
   e. Posaconazole 200 mg po tid

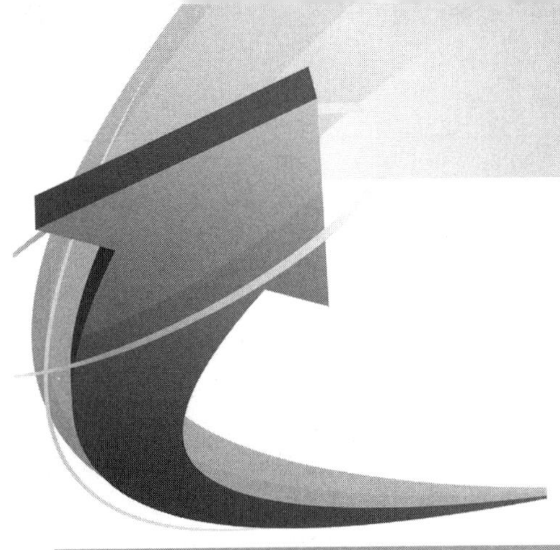

CASE 1.21
Severe Sepsis | Level 3

Demographics

PATIENT NAME: Joanna Johnson

AGE: 62

SEX: Female

HEIGHT: 5′5″

WEIGHT: 80 kg

RACE: White

ALLERGIES: NKDA

CHIEF COMPLAINT: J. J. presents to the ED complaining of pain, burning in her chest, and difficulty breathing.

HISTORY OF PRESENT ILLNESS: J. J. states that she has felt ill for the last 8 to 9 days. She presented to the ED 2 days ago and was given a prescription for a pain medication, a sedative, and an antibiotic. She has not been able to keep the oral medications down. She presents to the ED today with fever, chills, and sweats. A blood gas performed in ED reports a pO_2 of 77 mm Hg on room air. She has no previous history of pulmonary disease.

REVIEW OF SYSTEMS: Patient has no previous history of cardiac disease, pulmonary disease, kidney disease, or diabetes. Other than her recent respiratory tract disorder, her only complaint is diarrhea, which has persisted over the last couple of days.

PAST MEDICAL HISTORY: Past medical history is significant only for hypertension, which was diagnosed last year. According to the patient's daughter, she does have frequent headaches for which she takes about 25 Excedrin Extra Strength tablets every month.

SOCIAL HISTORY: She drinks a glass of wine occasionally and denies smoking.

FAMILY HISTORY: Noncontributory

Physical Examination

GEN: Alert and oriented yet appears tired and is quite dyspneic; extremities pale and mottled

VS: T 96.6°F, HR 115 bpm, RR 40 rpm, BP 80/50 mm Hg, O_2 sat 88%

Lungs: Bilateral rhonchi with decreased breath sounds in the right quadrant

CV: Tachycardia with a regular rhythm

Urine Output: 25 mL/hr over the last 2 hours

Laboratory and Diagnostic Tests

Sodium: 134 mEq/L

Potassium: 5.5 mEq/L

Chloride: 105 mEq/L

CO_2 Content: 13 mEq/L

BUN: 52 mg/dL

Serum Creatinine: 4.1 mg/dL

Glucose: 215 mg/dL

Hemoglobin: 13.8 g/dL

Hematocrit: 41%

Platelets: 188,000 cells/mm^3

WBC: 4,400 cells/mm^3

PMNs: 7%, bands 73%

Arterial Blood Gases (prior to intubation): pH 7.19, PaO_2 80 mm Hg, pCO_2 46 mm Hg, O_2 sat 88.9%, bicarbonate 17 mEq/L, FiO_2 15 L/min, base excess –9.8

Chest X-ray: Bilateral effusions with bibasilar consolidation

Cardiac Enzymes: CK 217 international units/L (elevated), CKMB 5.8 international units/L (elevated), troponin 2.6 ng/mL (elevated)

ECG: ST segment elevation

Diagnosis

Severe sepsis

Medication Record

Medications Prior to Admission

Atenolol 50 mg po daily

Conjugated estrogens (0.625 mg)/medroxyprogesterone (2.5 mg) one po daily

Levofloxacin 750 mg po daily

Zaleplon 10 mg po at bedtime

Acetaminophen with codeine 300 mg/30 mg 1 tablet q 6 hr prn moderate pain

Initial Inpatient Medication Profile

Ceftriaxone 2 g IVPB q 24 hr

Azithromycin 500 mg IVPB q 24 hr

Famotidine 20 mg IVP q 12 hr

Sodium bicarbonate 50 mEq IVP × 2

Morphine 1–4 mg IVP q 2 hr prn

Lactated Ringer's continuous infusion at 150 mL/hr

Midazolam 1 mg IVP × 1

Norepinephrine continuous infusion at 10 mcg/kg/min

Normal saline infusion wide open

D5NS infusion at 200 mL/hr

SELF-ASSESSMENT QUESTIONS

1. Describe the pathophysiology of severe sepsis.
2. On rounds in the ICU, the medical team asks you for your recommendations on whether J. J. should be placed on steroids for treating severe sepsis. What is your response?
3. The attending physician informs you that J. J.'s lactate level is 5.5 mmol/L. She asks you for your opinion on initial resuscitation goals for this patient. Based on the 2012 sepsis and septic shock guidelines, what is your response?
4. According to the 2012 sepsis and septic shock guidelines, what would be the best initial fluid resuscitation regimen (fluid type and amount) for J. J.?
5. It is postulated that J. J.'s myocardial infarction may have been a result of sepsis-induced hypotension. How is the treatment of her severe sepsis impacted by her myocardial infarction?
6. J. J.'s culture result from the bronchoscopy wash comes back reporting 4+ group A *Streptococcus*. Her antibiotics are changed from ceftriaxone to penicillin G 2 million units IVPB every 6 hours and clindamycin 900 mg IVPB every 8 hours. What is the rationale for using clindamycin in this situation, and what is an appropriate duration of antibiotic therapy?

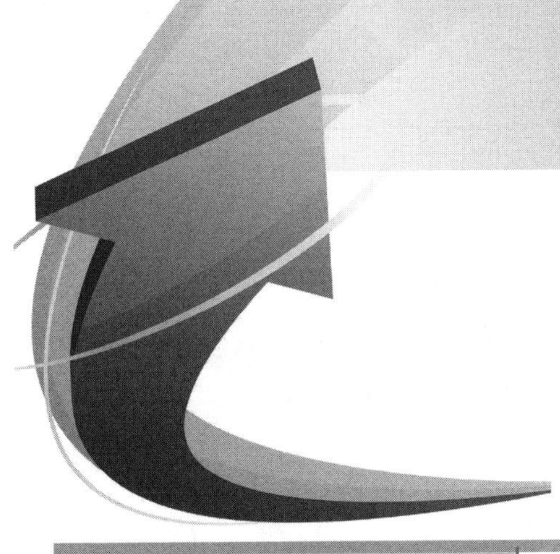

CASE 1.22
Septic Shock | Level 3

Demographics

PATIENT NAME: Jill Shay

AGE: 64

SEX: Female

HEIGHT: 5′5″

WEIGHT: 84 kg

RACE: Caucasian

ALLERGIES: Sulfa (hives)

CHIEF COMPLAINT: J. S. is a 64-year-old white female who presented to the ED complaining of increasing abdominal pain over the last 3 days. Besides the pain, she also complains of nausea and vomiting for the last 48 hours.

HISTORY OF PRESENT ILLNESS: J. S. was in her usual state of health up until 3 days ago. She awoke in the middle of the night due to acute abdominal pain and cramping. She took an H_2 blocker without relief. The pain continued over the next day and a half. In the last 12 hours, the pain has intensified, and she has not been able to keep anything down. At the time of presentation to the ED, J. S. was febrile and diaphoretic. She had severe lower right quadrant pain with rebound and guarding. She was evaluated by surgery for suspected appendicitis. J. S. underwent an emergency appendectomy. During surgery, she was found to have a perforated appendix with diffuse peritonitis; she became acutely hypotensive and required large volumes of fluid replacement. Postoperatively, she was transferred to the intensive care unit. She is intubated and continues to be hypotensive despite receiving 2 L of normal saline over the last 4 hours.

REVIEW OF SYSTEMS: Noncontributory except for physical exam findings

PAST MEDICAL HISTORY: 10-year history of HTN, treated with various antihypertensives; diagnosed with breast cancer 3 years ago and underwent a left mastectomy with subsequent radiation therapy

SOCIAL HISTORY: 40 pack-per-year history of smoking

FAMILY HISTORY: Noncontributory

Physical Examination

Gen: 64-year-old female who is intubated, diaphoretic, and in significant distress; pulmonary artery and arterial lines are in place

VS: BP (S/D/M) 70/50/57 mm Hg, HR 120 bpm, RR 20 rpm, T 103°F, Wt 84 kg

Hemodynamic Parameters: CO 8 L/min (normal 4–7), CI 3.5 L/min/m^2 (normal 2.5–4.2), PCWP 10 mm Hg (normal 5–12), CVP 4 mm Hg (normal 8–12), SVR 530 dyne/sec/cm^{-5} (normal 800–1,440)

Lungs: Reduced breath sounds bilaterally

Urine Output: 30 mL/hr over the last 2 hr

Laboratory and Diagnostic Tests

Sodium: 132 mEq/L

Potassium: 5.1 mEq/L

Chloride: 105 mEq/L

CO_2 Content: 22 mEq/L

BUN: 30 mg/dL

Serum Creatinine: 2.1 mg/dL

Glucose: 120 mg/dL

Hemoglobin: 12.2 g/dL

Hematocrit: 32%

Platelets: 110,000 cells/mm^3

WBC: 20,000 cells/mm^3

PMNs: 42%, bands 9%

Arterial Blood Gases (fraction of inspired oxygen 60%): pH 7.29, PaO_2 100 mm Hg, $PaCO_2$ 42 mm Hg, bicarbonate (HCO_3) 19 mEq/L

Diagnosis

Septic shock

Medication Record

Medications Prior to Admission

Hydrochlorothiazide 50 mg po daily

Atenolol 50 mg po daily

Aspirin 81 mg po daily

Atorvastatin 20 mg po daily

Lisinopril 20 mg po daily

Initial Inpatient Medication Profile

Heparin 5,000 units SC q 12 hr

Furosemide 40 mg IVP q 12 hr

Piperacillin/tazobactam 4.5 g IVPB q 6 hr

Gentamicin 60 mg IVPB q 12 hr

Pantoprazole 40 mg IVP q 24 hr

Morphine 1–4 mg IVP q 1–2 hr

Base fluids of D5LR/50 mEq sodium bicarbonate at 200 mL/hr

SELF-ASSESSMENT QUESTIONS

1. Based on the 2012 sepsis and septic shock guidelines for early goal-directed therapy, what is the most appropriate treatment plan at this time for J. S.?
2. Appropriate antimicrobial therapy continues to play a prominent role in the treatment of severe sepsis. Pharmacists can significantly impact outcomes from sepsis through their appropriate use. According to the 2012 sepsis and septic shock guidelines, appropriate antimicrobial therapy should be initiated within what time frame after recognition of septic shock?
3. When should de-escalation to the most appropriate single agent be done after culture and sensitivity data are reported?
4. What are ways that an antimicrobial stewardship team could benefit the care of J. S.?
5. In evaluating whether to use normal saline or albumin for the fluid resuscitation in J. S., the medical team asks you for your recommendations. Based on your analysis of the literature, what should your response be?
6. After fluid resuscitation, J. S. has the following hemodynamic parameters: mean arterial pressure 55 mm Hg, CVP 10 mm Hg, and cardiac index 3.0 L/min/m^2. The decision is made to administer a vasopressor. According to the 2012 consensus guidelines, what is the first choice therapy to administer in J. S.?

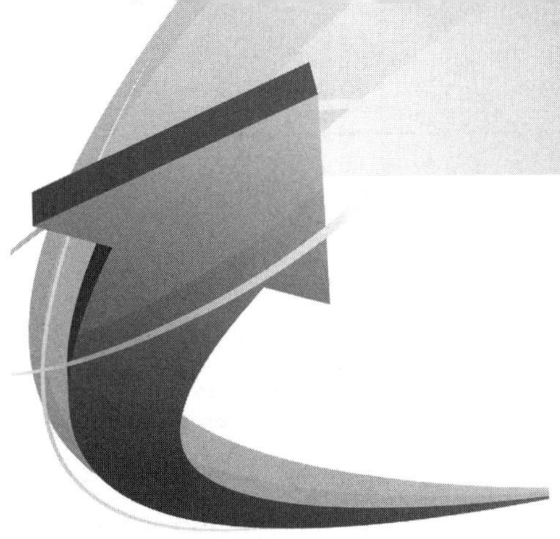

CASE 1.23
Complicated Urinary Tract Infection—Geriatric | Level 1

Demographics

PATIENT NAME: Jeffery Montgomery

AGE: 78

SEX: Male

HEIGHT: 5′10″

WEIGHT: 66 kg

RACE: White

ALLERGIES: Penicillin (rash)

CHIEF COMPLAINT: J. M. is a 78-year-old male who was admitted to the hospital from an area nursing home with fever, chills, vomiting, and flank pain.

HISTORY OF PRESENT ILLNESS: The patient was in his normal state of health until 48 hours prior to admission to the hospital when he started experiencing fevers to 102°F associated with shaking, chills, vomiting, and flank pain. He was seen by the nursing home physician the evening prior to admission and was given a single IM dose of ceftriaxone 1 g. The patient was transferred to the hospital this morning due to continued fever, chills, vomiting, and flank pain.

REVIEW OF SYSTEMS: Fever, chills, vomiting, and flank pain

PAST MEDICAL HISTORY: J. M. had a stroke with residual hemiparesis 3 years ago and has been wheelchair-bound since that time. In addition, he often requires catheterization to facilitate urination. The patient also has benign prostatic hypertrophy, HTN, HF, and glaucoma, which are all controlled with medication.

SOCIAL HISTORY: Noncontributory

FAMILY HISTORY: Noncontributory

Physical Examination

GEN: Pale, ill-looking, thin white male with poor skin turgor

VS: BP 92/65 mm Hg, HR 100 bpm, RR 22 rpm, T 39.5°C, Wt 66 kg

HEENT: PERRLA, oral cavity is dry

Chest: Equal shallow breath sounds, tachypneic, tachycardic

Neuro: Not easily arousable, disoriented to place and time

Back/Abd: Costovertebral angle tenderness, suprapubic tenderness

GU: Foley catheter in place

Laboratory and Diagnostic Tests

Sodium: 146 mEq/L

Potassium: 4.4 mEq/L

Chloride: 105 mEq/L

CO_2 Content: 25 mEq/L

BUN: 35 mg/dL

Serum Creatinine: 1.8 mg/dL

Glucose: 66 mg/dL

Hemoglobin: 13 g/dL

Hematocrit: 39%

Platelets: 225,000 cells/mm^3

WBC: 18,000 cells/mm^3 with 80% neutrophils, 8% bands, 10% lymphocytes, and 2% monocytes

Urinalysis (urine obtained from Foley catheter): Appearance amber-colored, cloudy, specific gravity 1.030, pH 6.5, WBC 20–25 cells/hpf, RBC 2–5 cells/hpf, protein negative, glucose negative, ketones trace, nitrite positive, leukocyte esterase positive, bacteria many

Urine Culture: 100,000 cfu/mL gram-negative rods, identification pending

Blood Culture: Gram-negative rods, identification pending

Diagnosis

Urinary tract infection (UTI)

Medication Record

Furosemide 40 mg po daily

Timolol 0.5% 1 gtt OU bid

Doxazosin 1 mg po daily

Accupril 10 mg po bid

MVI 1 po daily

Ceftriaxone 1 g IM × 1 yesterday

SELF-ASSESSMENT QUESTIONS

1. What risk factors contribute to the development of a complicated UTI in J. M., and what potential pathogens could result in the complicated UTI/urosepsis in J. M.?
2. Based on the initial Gram stain results from the urine and blood cultures, which of the following antibiotics is most appropriate for the empiric treatment of J. M.'s complicated UTI?
   a. Cefepime IV
   b. Ertapenem IV
   c. Oral TMP/SMX DS
   d. Ampicillin IV
   e. Oral doxycycline
3. The following day, the patient's fever and mental status improved, and the results of the urine and blood cultures and susceptibility results yield *Escherichia coli* susceptible to TMP/SMX, ampicillin/sulbactam, piperacillin/tazobactam, cefazolin, ceftriaxone, cefepime, imipenem, meropenem, levofloxacin, and tobramycin. Which of the following antibiotic regimens should be used for the continued treatment of J. M.'s infection (as directed therapy)?
   a. Cefepime 2 g IVPB q 24 hr
   b. Meropenem 1 g IVPB q 12 hr
   c. Cefazolin 1 g IVPB q 12 hr
   d. Tobramycin 400 mg IVPB q 24 hr
   e. Aztreonam 1 g IVPB q 8 hr
4. What is the recommended duration of antibiotic therapy for a patient with a complicated UTI, such as urosepsis and/or pyelonephritis?
5. Which of the following statements regarding urinary catheter use is ***false*** with regard to the development of UTIs?
   a. Urinary catheters do not increase the risk of developing UTIs.
   b. Bacteria may be introduced directly into the bladder during catheterization of the urinary tract.

c. The longer the patient has a urinary catheter, the greater the chance of developing a UTI.

d. In patients with long-term urinary catheters who develop symptomatic UTIs, replacement of the urinary catheter may decrease the incidence of reinfection.

e. Antibiotic prophylaxis is not recommended in patients with long-term indwelling catheters to prevent the development of UTIs because it may lead to the emergence of resistant bacteria.

6. Which of the following pharmacologic and nonpharmacologic measures can be recommended in the prevention and management of UTIs in J. M.?

   a. Cranberry juice has been conclusively shown to decrease the incidence of UTIs in males.

   b. Phenazopyridine should be recommended to all patients with UTIs to provide symptomatic relief of pain and burning on urination.

   c. The use of a condom catheter or intermittent bladder catheterization should be considered in males who require urinary catheterization to decrease the rate of UTIs.

   d. Prophylactic antibiotic therapy, given systemically or by bladder irrigation, should be routinely administered during urinary catheter insertion to decrease the risk of catheter-associated UTIs.

   e. Long-term suppressive antibiotic therapy should be given to all patients with recurrent UTIs to decrease the occurrence of future UTIs.

CASE 1.24
Urinary Tract Infection—Pediatric | Level 1

Demographics

PATIENT NAME: Michael Williams

AGE: 5

SEX: Male

HEIGHT: 4′0″

WEIGHT: 20 kg

RACE: African American

ALLERGIES: NKDA

CHIEF COMPLAINT: M. W. is a 5-year-old African-American boy who presents to the ED with complaints of burning on urination.

HISTORY OF PRESENT ILLNESS: M. W. started complaining of burning on urination 1.5 days ago. Yesterday, his temperature spiked to 101.4°F. He is not eating as usual and doesn't want to drink as he is hesitant to urinate.

REVIEW OF SYSTEMS: Fever present; complaining of burning on urination

PAST MEDICAL HISTORY: Bilateral kidney stones—12 months ago; hydronephrosis—12 months ago; generalized tonic-clonic seizure disorder—diagnosed at 2 years of age

SOCIAL HISTORY: Attends kindergarten 5 days per week, day care after school

FAMILY HISTORY: Mother and father—alive and in good health

Physical Examination

GEN: Well-nourished, healthy-appearing child

VS: BP 100/60 mm Hg, HR 100 bpm, RR 20 rpm, T 38.5°C, Wt 20 kg

ABD: Nontender, nondistended, bowel sounds present

GU: No abnormalities or deformities; foul-smelling, straw-colored, cloudy urine

Laboratory and Diagnostic Tests

Sodium: 145 mEq/L

Potassium: 4 mEq/L

Chloride: 101 mEq/L

CO_2 Content: 22 mEq/L

BUN: 7 mg/dL

Serum Creatinine: 0.5 mg/dL

Glucose: 100 mg/dL

UA: Nitrite (+), LE (+), WBC 10–50, RBC 1–4, many bacteria

Urine Culture: *E. coli*; susceptibilities pending

Diagnosis

Urinary tract infection (UTI)

Medication Record

Home Medications

Levetiracetam 500 mg po bid

Pediatric chewable multivitamin 1 tablet po daily

Past Medications

12 months ago: Ceftin 250 mg/5 mL suspension, 1 tsp po bid

3 months ago: Amoxicillin 400 mg/5 mL suspension, 2 tsp po bid

1 month ago: Ciprofloxacin 250 mg/5 mL suspension, 1 tsp po bid

Inpatient Medication Record

Ceftriaxone 1 g IV q 24 hr

Levetiracetam 500 mg po bid

SELF-ASSESSMENT QUESTIONS

1. What is a risk factor for M. W. developing a UTI due to an extended-spectrum beta-lactamase-producing (ESBL) organism? What organisms, other than *Escherichia coli*, are likely to produce an ESBL?
2. According to the antibiogram, what is the likelihood that the organism causing M. W.'s UTI is resistant to amoxicillin?
3. According to the antibiogram, there is a 30% likelihood that the organism causing M. W.'s UTI ________.
   a. Produces an extended-spectrum beta-lactamase
   b. Has mutations in the folate synthesis enzymes
   c. Has a mutation in the 30S ribosomal subunit
   d. Produces an aminoglycoside-modifying enzyme
   e. Produces a fluoroquinolone efflux pump
4. Why should imipenem/cilastatin be avoided for use in M. W.?
5. According to the antibiogram, what is the likelihood that the organism causing M. W.'s UTI is resistant to ceftriaxone?
6. The hospital antibiogram can be used to ________.
   a. Select antibiotic therapy after culture and susceptibilities have returned
   b. Track the use of broad-spectrum antibiotics in a healthcare system
   c. Monitor trends in antimicrobial resistance patterns over time

ANTIBIOGRAM						
	Ampicillin	**Gentamicin**	**Cefotaxime**	**Ciprofloxacin**	**Imipenem**	**TMP/SMX**
E. cloacae	40	50	40	90	95	50
E. coli	55	85	90	80	99	70
P. aeruginosa	—	60	—	70	60	—
E. faecalis	90	—	—	—	90	—
E. faecium	45	—	—	—	40	—

d. Guide empiric antiviral therapy during influenza season
e. Calculate the percentage of UTIs caused by *E. coli*.

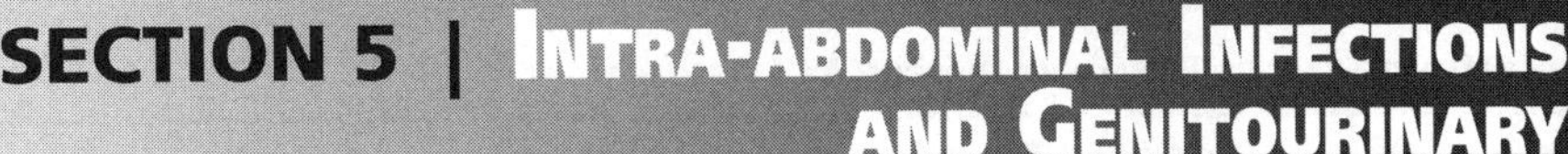

CASE 1.25
Uncomplicated Urinary Tract Infection | Level 2

Demographics

PATIENT NAME: Karen Aldridge

AGE: 23

SEX: Female

HEIGHT: 5′6″

WEIGHT: 65 kg

RACE: Caucasian

ALLERGIES: Shellfish (swollen lips), amoxicillin (rash)

CHIEF COMPLAINT: K. A. is a 23-year-old female who presents to the ambulatory care clinic with complaints of pain and burning on urination, with an increased need to urinate for the past 3 days.

HISTORY OF PRESENT ILLNESS: K. A. first noticed pain and burning with urination about 3 days ago. Since then, she has noticed an increased need to urinate and has made about 10 trips to the bathroom to urinate for the past 2 days. She has been drinking cranberry juice since her symptoms began but has not experienced any relief in her symptoms.

REVIEW OF SYSTEMS: Pain and burning on urination, with increased urinary frequency

PAST MEDICAL HISTORY: K. A. was diagnosed with acute uncomplicated cystitis 6 months earlier at the student health clinic just before she graduated from college. She was given a 3-day course of an antibiotic but cannot recall its name. She has not seen a physician in the recent past for any specific medical conditions, but she had obtained a prescription for birth control pills from the student health center before graduating. She recently started a new job that provides medical insurance, but she does not have prescription benefits. Other past medical history includes a tonsillectomy at the age of 7 years and a fractured forearm when she was a freshman in college.

SOCIAL HISTORY: Tobacco use—none; alcohol use—socially; sexually active with a single partner for the past 12 months

FAMILY HISTORY: Mother and father—alive; father—mild HTN (controlled with diet and exercise)

Physical Examination

Gen: WDWN young white female with slight suprapubic tenderness on examination; does not have costovertebral angle tenderness

VS: BP 128/62 mm Hg, HR 70 bpm, RR 12 rpm, T 37.5°C, Wt 65 kg

Laboratory and Diagnostic Tests

Urinalysis: From a midstream, clean-catch urine specimen, appearance straw-colored, specific gravity 1.020, pH 6.5, glucose negative, ketones negative, protein negative, nitrite positive, leukocyte esterase positive, WBC 10–15 cells/hpf, RBC 0–2 cells/hpf, bacteria many, hCG negative

Diagnosis

Urinary tract infection (UTI)

Medication Record

Gianvi 1 tablet po daily

SELF-ASSESSMENT QUESTIONS

1. What are known risk factors for the development of a UTI? What symptoms, physical exam findings, and laboratory findings are suggestive of acute uncomplicated cystitis in this patient? What bacteria is the most common cause of acute uncomplicated cystitis in females?
2. Which of the following pharmacologic and nonpharmacologic measures can be recommended in the management of UTIs in K. A.?
   a. Cranberry juice has been conclusively shown to decrease the incidence of UTIs in females.
   b. Phenazopyridine should be recommended to all patients with UTIs to provide symptomatic relief of pain and burning on urination.
   c. In women who experience repeated symptomatic UTIs associated with sexual activity, voiding after intercourse may help prevent infection.
   d. The use of spermicide-coated condoms during sexual intercourse may decrease the occurrence of UTIs.
   e. Long-term suppressive antibiotic therapy should be given to all patients with recurrent UTIs to decrease the occurrence of future UTIs.
3. A first-year medical resident asks you for a recommendation regarding the appropriate antibiotic treatment for this patient's acute uncomplicated cystitis. The clinic outpatient antibiogram demonstrates that 82% of *Escherichia coli* isolates are susceptible to TMP/SMX. Which of the following regimens would be most appropriate to treat this patient's UTI?
   a. Amoxicillin 500 mg po q 8 hr for 7 days
   b. Azithromycin 1 g po as a single dose
   c. Tetracycline 250 mg po q 6 hr for 7 days
   d. TMP/SMX 1 DS tablet po bid for 3 days
   e. Levofloxacin 250 mg po daily for 7 days
4. If the results of the patient's urine hCG had been positive, which antibiotic class should not be used in any trimester during pregnancy because of potential harm to the unborn fetus?
5. What antibiotic would be most appropriate to treat a nonpregnant female patient with acute uncomplicated cystitis who is allergic to sulfonamide antibiotics?
   a. Ceftriaxone 1 g IV daily
   b. Doxycycline 100 mg po bid
   c. Ciprofloxacin 250 mg po bid
   d. Nitrofurantoin monohydrate/macrocrystals 100 mg po bid
   e. Azithromycin 1 g po as a single dose
6. K. A. returns to the ambulatory clinic several months later with signs and symptoms of another episode of acute uncomplicated cystitis. Which of the following treatment strategies would be most appropriate for this patient?
   a. The current infection is most likely due to a resistant organism so the patient should be treated with a 14-day course of an oral fluoroquinolone, such as levofloxacin.
   b. The current infection is most likely due to reinfection and should be treated with a 14-day course of TMP/SMX.
   c. Due to K. A.'s frequent occurrences of UTIs (three episodes within 1 year), she should be treated for this episode of acute uncom-

plicated cystitis with TMP/SMX DS 1 tablet po bid for 3 days and counseled about lifestyle modifications in an attempt to decrease the recurrence of infection.

d. The patient should receive a 10-day course of IV ceftriaxone 1 g IV daily because oral therapy has been ineffective in the treatment of her infections.

e. The patient's birth control should be switched to spermicide-coated condoms to minimize the development of recurrent UTIs.

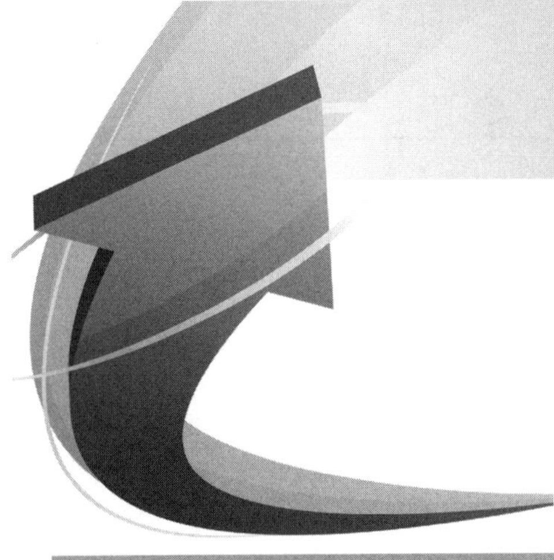

CASE 1.26
Intra-abdominal Infection | Level 3

Demographics

PATIENT NAME: Patricia Hinds

AGE: 67

SEX: Female

HEIGHT: 5′5″

WEIGHT: 155 lb

RACE: Caucasian

ALLERGIES: Morphine (itching)

CHIEF COMPLAINT: P. H. is a 67-year-old female presenting to the ED with abdominal pain for several days.

HISTORY OF ILLNESS: P. H. states that the pain began 6 days ago when she was experiencing diarrhea and vomiting. She thought she had acquired a stomach bug from her granddaughter. The diarrhea lasted 3 days, but the vomiting and pain have persisted. She has a poor appetite and vomits when she tries to eat. P. H. describes her pain in the lower abdomen region and rates her pain a 10 out of 10. She states that she has never experienced any pain like this before. Her last bowel movement was 2 days ago, and she has not passed gas today. P. H. denies chest pain and shortness of breath.

REVIEW OF SYSTEMS: + abdominal pain; + N/V/D; no other systems reviewed

PAST MEDICAL HISTORY: Asthma; HTN; hyperlipidemia; coronary artery disease—two stents placed, most recent 2 years ago; cholecystectomy; hysterectomy

SOCIAL HISTORY: Denies alcohol or tobacco use; no illicit drug use

FAMILY HISTORY: Mother—ulcerative colitis; father—thyroid cancer; sister—rheumatoid arthritis

IMMUNIZATION HISTORY: Up-to-date as of 2 years ago

Physical Examination

Gen: Alert and oriented; moderate distress

VS: Ht 5′5″, Wt 155 lb, HR 90 bpm, RR 18 rpm, T 98.9°F, BP 108/71 mm Hg, O_2 sat 94% on room air

HEENT: EOMI, PERRLA

Chest: Lungs CTA, normal breath sounds, no respiratory distress, heart RRR

Abd: Guarding, rebound, distended, diffuse tenderness and hypoactive BS

Ext: Unremarkable

Laboratory and Diagnostic Tests

Sodium: 135 mEq/L

Potassium: 3.1 mEq/L

Chloride: 97 mEq/L

CO_2 Content: 29 mEq/L

BUN: 12 mg/dL

Serum Creatinine: 1.2 mg/dL

Glucose: 102 mg/dL

Calcium: 8.5 mc/dL

AST: 14 international units/L

ALT: 13 international units/L

ALP: 58 international units/L

Total Protein: 7.1 g/dL

Albumin: 3.7 g/dL

Lipase: 55 units/L

CBC: WBC 17,900 cells/mm^3, 85% PMNs, 13% lymphocytes, 2% monocytes, 0% eosinophils, 0% basophils

Hemoglobin: 13.9 g/dL

Hematocrit: 42%

Platelets: 312,000 cells/mm^3

CRP: 5 mg/dL

Urinalysis: Appearance yellow, clear, specific gravity 1.020, pH 8.0, WBC 2 cells/hpf, RBC 2 cells/hpf, protein 1+ (high), glucose negative, ketones 1+ (high), nitrite negative, urobilinogen 4.0 (high), leukocyte esterase negative

CT Abd: Diverticulitis of the colon with perforation and associated air bubble in pericolonic fat

Diagnosis

Diverticulitis

Medication Record

Home Medications

Ranexa 500 mg po daily

Clopidogrel 75 mg po daily

Aspirin 325 mg po daily

Lisinopril 20 mg po daily

Nebivolol 10 mg po daily

Nitroglycerin 1 tablet sublingually prn as directed

Pravastatin 40 mg po daily

Fluticasone/salmeterol 115 mcg/21 mcg, 2 puffs bid

Inpatient Medications

Continue home medications

Piperacillin/tazobactam 3.375 g IVPB q 6 hr

Metronidazole 500 mg IVPB q 6 hr

LOCAL INSTITUTION'S ANTIBIOGRAM

	Gram Negative								Gram Positive					
Organism	*E. cloacae*	*E. coli*	*K. oxytoca*	*K. pneumoniae*	*P. aeruginosa*	*P. mirabilis*	*S. maltophilia*	*S. marcescens*	*E. faecalis*	*E. faecium*	*S. epidermidis*	*S. haemolyticus*	*S. aureus* (MSSA)	*S. aureus* (MRSA)
# of isolates	**80**	**704**	**42**	**224**	**224**	**98**	**33**	**44**	**318**	**87**	**190**	***21**	**267**	**345**
Ampicillin		43				89			99					
Ampicillin/ sulbactam		47	52	83		96								
Cefazolin		81		92		92							100	
Cefepime	92	89	100	95	86	100		100						
Ceftriaxone	70	88	98	95		100		98						
Cefuroxime		83	86	85		97								
Daptomycin											99	100	100	100
Doripenem	100	100	100	100	91	98		100						
Erythromycin													62	
Gentamicin	92	86	98	97	85	90		100			74	71	99	99
Imipenem	100	100	100	100	85	99		100						
Levofloxacin	88	61	100	96	76	61	79	95	71				87	
Linezolid										100	98	95	100	100
Oxacillin													100	
Penicillin									99				22	
Piperacillin/ tazobactam	79	98	95	96	90	100		98						
Rifampin									62		98	100	100	198
Tetracycline	88		93	84						24	83		93	96
Tobramycin	91	85	100	96	95	92		98						
Trimethoprim/ sulfamethoxazole	86	68	98	91		74	100	98			47		100	98
Vancomycin									97	33	100	100	100	100

Organism	**# of isolates**	**Ceftriaxone (meningitis)**	**Ceftriaxone (non-meningitis)**	**Erythromycin**	**Levofloxacin**	**Penicillin**	**Vancomycin**
Streptococcus pneumoniae	54	89	98	43	98	43	100

SELF-ASSESSMENT QUESTIONS

1. What is the optimal time frame in which antibiotics should be administered to a patient with an intra-abdominal infection?
2. The medical resident asks you if blood cultures should be ordered and drawn to identify the potential pathogen in P. H. What is the best response to the resident?
3. What recommendations would you make, if any, for the empiric antibiotic regimen that has been initiated for P. H.?
4. What if the physician had initiated levofloxacin and metronidazole for empiric therapy for P. H.? What recommendations would you make, if any, for the antibiotic regimen?
5. What treatment duration is best to recommend for P. H.?
6. You have been asked to participate in the new antimicrobial stewardship program at the hospital. Per the IDSA guidelines, what strategies could the program consider to initiate based on hospital resources?

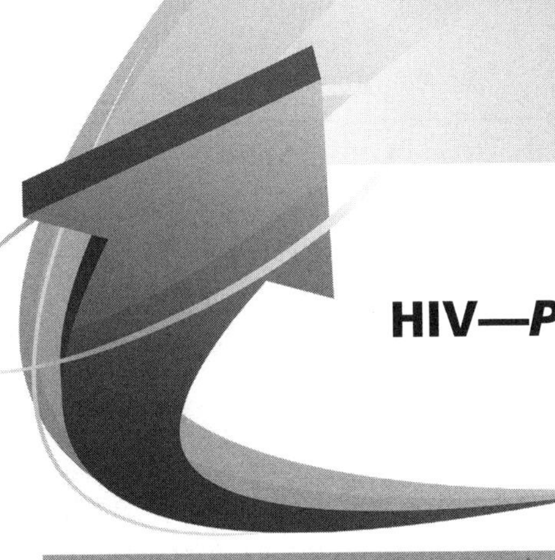

CASE 1.27
HIV—*Pneumocystis jirovecii* Pneumonia | Level 2

Demographics

PATIENT NAME: Jacob Cash

AGE: 36

SEX: Male

HEIGHT: 5′11″

WEIGHT: 143 lb

RACE: White

ALLERGIES: NKDA

CHIEF COMPLAINT: J. C. is a 36-year-old man admitted to the hospital 4 days ago for fever, productive cough, shortness of breath, and fatigue. Chest x-ray and symptoms were suggestive of *Pneumocystis jirovecii* pneumonia (PCP), so consent was obtained for an HIV antibody test, which was positive. J. C. is responding to treatment for PCP and will complete therapy (3 weeks total) as an outpatient. He is initiating antiretroviral therapy today, anticipating discharge from the hospital tomorrow.

HISTORY OF PRESENT ILLNESS: J. C. presented to the ED 4 days ago when he was unable to climb one flight of stairs in his home without becoming extremely short of breath. He reported a 2-week history of worsening cough, fatigue, and dyspnea on exertion. He also reported fevers to 101°F for 3 days prior to admission and an unintentional 15-lb weight loss over the past 3 months. In the ED, his oxygen saturation was 86% on room air.

REVIEW OF SYSTEMS: More comfortable, less shortness of breath

PAST MEDICAL HISTORY: J. C. had not been tested for HIV prior to this admission. He has a history of genital HSV but has been otherwise healthy.

SOCIAL HISTORY: MSM; lives with his partner of 6 years; practices safe sex but admits to unprotected anal intercourse several years ago; family knows of his diagnosis and is supportive; tobacco use—none; alcohol use—1 to 2 glasses of wine with dinner each evening

FAMILY HISTORY: Parents and one sister—alive and in good health

Physical Examination

Gen: Thin, white male sitting up in bed in NAD

VS: Wt 65 kg, Ht 5′11″, BP 116/74 mm Hg, HR 70 bpm, T 99.4°F

Skin: Warm, pink with good turgor; possible fine macular rash starting on chest/neck

HEENT: PERRLA, ears and nose clear, oral cavity without lesions

Chest: Fine crackles and decreased breath sounds bilaterally

Abd: No tenderness or guarding, good bowel sounds

GU: WNL

Rect: WNL

Laboratory and Diagnostic Tests

Sodium: 133 mEq/L

Potassium: 4.2 mEq/L

Chloride: 104 mEq/L

CO_2 Content: 21 mEq/L

BUN: 20 mg/dL

Serum Creatinine: 0.9 mg/dL

Glucose: 96 mg/dL

Hemoglobin: 14.5 g/dL

Hematocrit: 44%

Platelets: 186,000 cells/mm^3

WBC: 10,600 cells/mm^3 with 78% PMNs, 18% lymphocytes, 2% monocytes, 2% eosinophils

Lymphocyte Subset Analysis: CD4 cells 69/mm^3, CD8 cells 230/mm^3

HIV Assays: ELISA positive, confirmed by Western blot

HIV RNA: 192,930 copies/mL

Chest X-ray: Diffuse interstitial pulmonary infiltrates

Induced Sputum: DFA stain positive for *Pneumocystis jirovecii*

Diagnosis

Pneumocystis jirovecii pneumonia

Medication Record

Inpatient Record

D5/0.45 NS 1,000 mL, infuse at 42 mL/hr

Sulfamethoxazole/trimethoprim 20 mL/500 mL D5W, infuse over 90 min q 8 hr

Acetaminophen 500 mg, 1–2 tablets po q 4–6 hr prn

Temazepam 15 mg po qpm

Tenofovir/emtricitabine (Truvada) 1 tablet po daily

Darunavir (Prezista) 800 mg po daily

Ritonavir (Norvir) 100 mg po daily

Diphenhydramine 25 mg, 1–2 tablets po q 6 hr prn

SELF-ASSESSMENT QUESTIONS

1. The physician wants to start sulfamethoxazole/trimethoprim. What is the best treatment regimen for J. C.?
2. What alternative regimen for the treatment of PCP may result in hemolysis if administered to a patient with glucose-6-phosphate dehydrogenase deficiency?
3. What is the primary role of ritonavir in J. C.'s regimen?
4. To deem the antiretroviral regimen a success, what should the plasma HIV RNA be at J. C.'s 2-month follow-up visit?
5. If J. C.'s work-up had revealed a PPD and a CXR consistent with active pulmonary tuberculosis, what antituberculous medication would be contraindicated with his antiretroviral regimen?
6. What is the most appropriate regimen for the prophylaxis of PCP, and how long should J. C. take it?

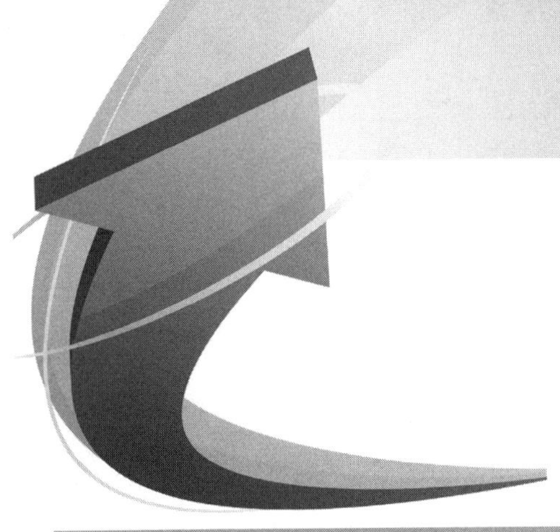

CASE 1.28
HIV Medication Management | Level 2

Demographics

PATIENT NAME: Paul Thomas

AGE: 25

SEX: Male

HEIGHT: 5′9″

WEIGHT: 68 kg

RACE: White

ALLERGIES: Sulfa (rash)

CHIEF COMPLAINT: P. T. is a 25-year-old man with HIV who returns to the outpatient HIV/AIDS clinic for his scheduled follow-up visit. P. T. reports that he has been doing well on his first and current antiretroviral regimen and is back to working full-time as a banker. With his busy daily schedule, he admits to missing two doses per week.

HISTORY OF PRESENT ILLNESS: P. T. was diagnosed as HIV-seropositive 18 months ago. At that time, his CD4 cell count was 247 cells/mm^3 and plasma HIV RNA was 135,590 copies/mL. Within a month of diagnosis, P. T. began this cART regimen. Subsequent monitoring has shown a steady increase in CD4 cell count to 442 cells/mm^3 with a drop in plasma HIV RNA to less than 50 copies/mL (both measured at his last visit 3 months ago). He is seen in the clinic for follow-up at regular 3-month intervals.

REVIEW OF SYSTEMS: No nausea/vomiting/diarrhea

PAST MEDICAL HISTORY: At the time of HIV diagnosis, P. T. had an episode of oral candidiasis. He has not had any opportunistic infections and rarely has symptoms associated with the virus. He was diagnosed with hypertension about 6 months ago, which is stable on antihypertensive therapy. He has a history of depression.

SOCIAL HISTORY: Bisexual male, currently in monogamous heterosexual relationship, uses condoms; tobacco use—none; alcohol use—one mixed drink or 1 to 2 glasses of wine per week

FAMILY HISTORY: Noncontributory

VACCINE HISTORY: Childhood series up-to-date; no vaccines since age 18

Physical Examination

Gen: WDWN male in NAD

VS: Wt 68 kg, Ht 5′9″, BP 124/80 mm Hg, HR 86 bpm, T 98.8°F

Skin: Supple, no lesions

HEENT: PERRLA, ears and nose clear, oral cavity without lesions

Chest: Clear to auscultation, good breath sounds

Abd: No tenderness or guarding, good bowel sounds

GU: WNL

Rect: Declined

Laboratory and Diagnostic Tests

Sodium: 140 mEq/L

Potassium: 4.0 mEq/L

Chloride: 101 mEq/L

CO_2 Content: 26 mEq/L

BUN: 12 mg/dL

Serum Creatinine: 0.7 mg/dL

Glucose: 88 mg/dL

Hemoglobin: 13.8 g/dL

Hematocrit: 40%

Platelets: 157,000 cells/mm^3

WBC: 7,200 cells/mm^3 with 64% neutrophils, 22% lymphocytes, 13% monocytes, 1% eosinophils

CD4 Cells: 180/mm^3

HIV RNA PCR: 102,240 copies/mL

HIV Genotype: Resistance to first-generation nonnucleoside reverse transcriptase inhibitors; HLAB5701 (+)

Tropism Assay: R5; G6PD deficient; toxoplasma IgG +; HAV Ab +; HBsAb +; HBsAg–; HBcAb–; HCV Ab–

Diagnosis

HIV medication management visit

Medication Record

Efavirenz 600 mg/tenofovir 300 mg/emtricitabine 200 mg po qhs

Hydrochlorothiazide 12.5 mg po daily

Citalopram 20 mg po daily

Multivitamin 1 tablet po daily

SELF-ASSESSMENT QUESTIONS

1. What ART must be avoided for treatment of this patient's HIV? What ART remains as options for this patient?
2. What is the most appropriate recommendation for P. T.'s opportunistic infection prophylaxis plan?
3. What is the most appropriate therapy for HIV for P. T. at this time?
   a. Change regimen to lamivudine, tenofovir, and efavirenz
   b. Change regimen to zidovudine, lamivudine, and tenofovir
   c. Change regimen to abacavir, lamivudine, darunavir, and ritonavir
   d. Change regimen to tenofovir, emtricitabine, and dolutegravir
   e. Change regimen to tenofovir, emtricitabine, and rilpivirine
4. A patient initiating therapy with efavirenz should be informed of the potential for what adverse effect?
   a. Jaundice
   b. Vivid dreams
   c. Skin hyperpigmentation
   d. Lipodystrophy
   e. Peripheral neuropathy
5. What vaccines are appropriate to administer to P. T. at this time?
6. Patients should be counseled to administer all of the following antiretroviral agents with a meal except ________.
   a. Rilpivirine
   b. Efavirenz
   c. Darunavir
   d. Elvitegravir
   e. Atazanavir

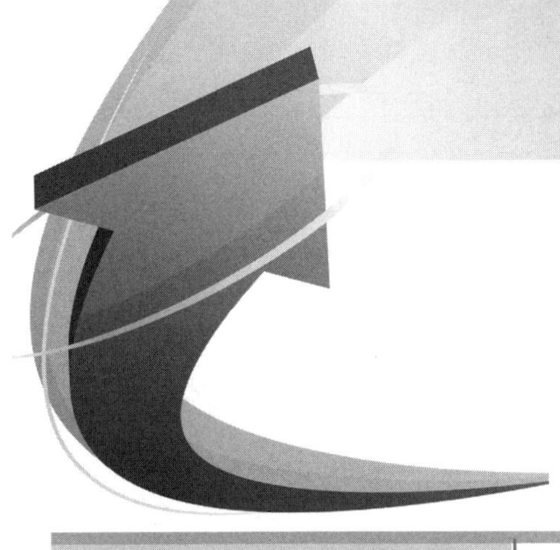

CASE 1.29
Vulvovaginal Candidiasis | Level 1

Demographics

PATIENT NAME: Lori Daniels

AGE: 27

SEX: Female

HEIGHT: 5′4″

WEIGHT: 135 lb

RACE: White

ALLERGIES: Fluoroquinolones (hives)

CHIEF COMPLAINT: L. D. complains of a thick, white vaginal discharge with intense itching and burning in the vaginal area.

HISTORY OF PRESENT ILLNESS: L. D.'s current symptoms began 5 days ago. Patient had sinusitis and finished up a course of Augmentin 4 days ago.

REVIEW OF SYSTEMS: Negative except for above

PAST MEDICAL HISTORY: Gravida 1, para 1; LMP was 16 days ago; occasional heartburn

SOCIAL HISTORY: Alcohol—rare; tobacco—none; occupation—elementary school teacher; married—one child, 3 years old

FAMILY HISTORY: Mother and father—alive and well

VACCINE HISTORY: Up-to-date

Physical Examination

GEN: Pleasant female in NAD

VS: BP 130/70 mm Hg, HR 68 bpm, T 37.1°C

PELVIC: White, malodorous vaginal discharge

Laboratory and Diagnostic Tests

Wet mount (KOH) reveals yeast

Diagnosis

Vulvovaginal candidiasis

Medication Record

Ortho-Novum 1/35, 1 tablet po daily

SELF-ASSESSMENT QUESTIONS

1. What is the most common cause of vulvovaginal candidiasis?
2. What are signs, symptoms, and risk factors of vulvovaginal candidiasis?
3. Over-the-counter (OTC) vaginal candidiasis products are appropriate for _______.
   a. Patients with similar symptoms who have had a previously diagnosed vaginal yeast infection
   b. Pregnant women
   c. Recurrent (more than four episodes per year) vaginal candidiasis
   d. Patients less than 12 years of age
   e. Patients with foul-smelling vaginal discharge
4. What are appropriate drug therapy options (nonprescription and prescription) for vulvovaginal candidiasis? Compare and contrast these agents.
5. What is the appropriate treatment duration for vulvovaginal candidiasis?
6. All of the following statements are appropriate counseling points for L. D. ***except*** _______.
   a. Signs and symptoms should improve in 48 to 72 hours.
   b. Common adverse effects associated with intravaginal antifungal products include vulvovaginal irritation, burning, and pruritus.
   c. Complete the full course of therapy.
   d. Stop using the medication if menstruation begins.
   e. Certain products are oil-based and may weaken a latex condom or diaphragm.

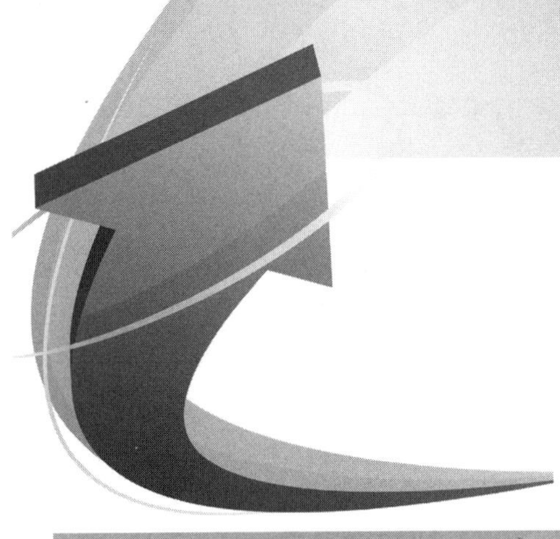

CASE 1.30
Disseminated Candidiasis | Level 3

Demographics

PATIENT NAME: Martha Barbary

AGE: 52

SEX: Female

HEIGHT: 5′2″

WEIGHT: 71.8 kg

RACE: White

ALLERGIES: Erythromycin (severe diarrhea)

CHIEF COMPLAINT: M. B. is a 52-year-old female who was admitted 15 days ago for a small bowel obstruction. She has remained in the surgical ICU for 15 days. M. B. is currently on vancomycin, meropenem, tobramycin, and fluconazole for nosocomial pneumonia and an MRSA wound infection. Her WBC count has been increasing over the past 3 days. This morning, she spiked a temperature to 103.4°F, and her blood pressure dropped to 85/46 mm Hg.

HISTORY OF PRESENT ILLNESS: M. B. was admitted 15 days ago for a small bowel obstruction. She underwent a small bowel resection on the day of admission. M. B. was emergently brought back to the operating room 4 days later with a perforation. She has subsequently had multiple other trips to the OR secondary to this perforation. M. B. developed an MRSA wound infection 7 days ago and was placed on vancomycin. She then developed nosocomial pneumonia 5 days ago and was placed on ceftazidime. Three days ago, her WBC increased, and her ceftazidime was discontinued, and she was placed on meropenem, tobramycin, and fluconazole. Today, her WBC is 32,000 with 62% segs and 18% bands. She is hypotensive and requiring 100% oxygen via mechanical ventilation. She has central venous access. M. B. has been in the surgical ICU since admission.

REVIEW OF SYSTEMS: Negative except as noted previously

PAST MEDICAL HISTORY: Arthritis, HTN × 8 years, and prediabetes (recently diagnosed); history of UTIs; gravida 3, para 3

SOCIAL HISTORY: Alcohol—none; tobacco—none; married × 22 years; three children—ages 16, 18, 21

Family History: Mother—HTN, hyperthyroidism; father—deceased 1997, MVA; brother—HTN, diabetes; sister—no known medical problems

Physical Examination

Gen: Critically ill female, intubated, in moderate distress

VS: BP 86/50 mm Hg, HR 132 bpm, RR 28 rpm, T 103.2°F, Wt 71.8 kg

HEENT: PERRLA, intubated, funduscopic exam is negative

Chest: Diminished breath sounds bilaterally, rales at both bases

Abd: Mild erythema around surgical incisions, colostomy pink, mild hepatomegaly

Ext: 2+ pitting edema, no rash

Lymph: No nodes

Laboratory and Diagnostic Tests

Sodium: 132 mEq/L

Potassium: 3.8 mEq/L

Chloride: 114 mEq/L

CO_2 Content: 22 mEq/L

BUN: 24 mg/dL

Serum Creatinine: 1.1 mg/dL

Glucose: 210 mg/dL

Hemoglobin: 11.1 g/dL

Hematocrit: 34%

Platelets: 372,000 cells/mm^3

WBC: 32,000 cells/mm^3 with 62% segs, 18% bands

CXR: Consolidation in both lower lobes, unchanged from prior exam

Micro: Blood cultures, negative × 2 days; sputum, 2+ yeast; urine, yeast

Diagnosis

Disseminated candidiasis

Medication Record

4/1 ampicillin/sulbactam 3 g IVPB q 6 hr

4/1 morphine sulfate prn

4/1 midazolam drip IV

4/4 TPN

4/8 vancomycin 1 g IVPB q 12 hr

4/8 levofloxacin 500 mg IVPB q 24 hr

4/8 metronidazole 500 mg IVPB q 8 hr

4/8 D/C ampicillin/sulbactam

4/10 ceftazidime 2 g q IV 8 hr

4/10 D/C levofloxacin

4/10 fluconazole 400 mg IV q 24 hr

4/13 meropenem 1 g IV q 8 hr

4/13 tobramycin 170 mg IV q 8 hr

4/13 D/C ceftazidime

4/13 D/C metronidazole

4/15 dopamine drip IV

SELF-ASSESSMENT QUESTIONS

1. What are risk factors for disseminated (systemic) candidiasis? What are M. B.'s risk factors?
2. What is the most appropriate antifungal agent for M. B. at this time?
3. Which species of *Candida* is intrinsically resistant to fluconazole?
4. A physician asks you for a recommendation for antifungal therapy. Upon review of patient information, you notice that the patient has a creatinine clearance of 15 mL/min. Which agent should be avoided in this patient?
   a. Liposomal amphotericin
   b. Voriconazole oral
   c. Anidulafungin IV
   d. Voriconazole IV
   e. Fluconazole oral
5. What agents would be considered appropriate empiric therapy if a non-*albicans Candida* species was suspected?
6. What antifungals are active against *Aspergillus* species?

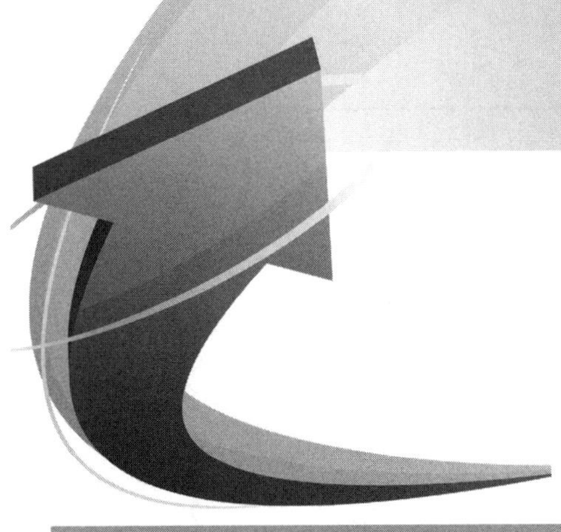

CASE 1.31
Lyme Disease | Level 1

Demographics

PATIENT NAME: Sarah Hunter

AGE: 32

SEX: Female

HEIGHT: 5′5″

WEIGHT: 145 lb

RACE: Caucasian

ALLERGIES: Latex

CHIEF COMPLAINT: S. H. is a 32-year-old woman who presented to the internal medicine clinic complaining of fatigue and joint pain. She states that she feels like she has the flu and is asking for a prescription.

HISTORY OF PRESENT ILLNESS: S. H. recently returned from camping in New Hampshire approximately 10 days ago, which is when she first felt very tired. The next morning she began to feel muscle aches and a headache. She thought that she was developing the flu and began to self-medicate with OTC strength ibuprofen with no success. Her husband noticed that she had a large red circular area on her back near the right shoulder. She then presented to the clinic for evaluation.

REVIEW OF SYSTEMS: Fatigue, muscle ache, and annular lesion

PAST MEDICAL HISTORY: Noncontributory

SOCIAL HISTORY: Tobacco use—yes; alcohol use—socially; sexually active with multiple partners over the past 12 years; now married with a 4-year-old son

FAMILY HISTORY: Mother—good health; father—died 3 years ago at age 59 from a heart attack; no siblings

VACCINE HISTORY: DTaP, polio, MMR completed series; chicken pox at age 3 years

Physical Examination

GEN: Well-developed, well-nourished young Caucasian female with fatigue, myalgia, and annular lesion on right shoulder

VS: BP 118/68 mm Hg, HR 86 bpm, RR 20 rpm, T 98.6°F, Wt 145 lb

HEENT: Within normal limits

Cardiac: Normal sinus rhythm

Chest: Right shoulder annular lesion with bright red borders warm to the touch (consistent with erythema migrans)

Ext: Normal range of motion, no joint swelling or erythema

Laboratory and Diagnostic Tests

<u>**Serum Chemistry**</u>

Sodium: 138 mEq/L

Potassium: 4.1 mEq/L

Chloride: 103 mEq/L

CO_2 Content: 26 mEq/L

BUN: 11 mg/dL

Serum Creatinine: 0.8 mg/dL

Glucose: 84 mg/dL

<u>**CBC with Differential**</u>

Hemoglobin: 11.7 g/dL

Hematocrit: 35%

Platelets: 278,000 cells/mm^3

WBC: 9,000 cells/mm^3 with 52% PMNs

<u>**Miscellaneous Results**</u>

CXR: Unremarkable

ESR: 45 mm/hr

ELISA: Positive

Pregnancy Test: Negative

Diagnosis

Lyme disease

Medication Record

Ethinyl estradiol 0.035 mg/ norgestimate 0.25 mg, 1 tablet po daily

SELF-ASSESSMENT QUESTIONS

1. What main risk factors does S. H. have for developing Lyme disease?
2. S. H.'s physical findings are most consistent with which stage of Lyme disease?
3. Which of S. H.'s lab results, besides ELISA, is most consistent with Lyme disease?
4. What would be the most appropriate treatment regimen for S. H., and what is the duration of treatment?
5. The most effective way for S. H. to prevent future episodes of Lyme disease would be ________.
   a. Ceftriaxone 1 g IM × 1 dose after prolonged outdoor activity
   b. Administration of the Lyme disease vaccine
   c. Application of tick repellent containing DEET to skin before outdoor activity
   d. Doxycycline 100 mg po bid during the summer months
   e. Azithromycin 1 g po weekly during the summer months
6. What immunizations does S. H. need at this time?

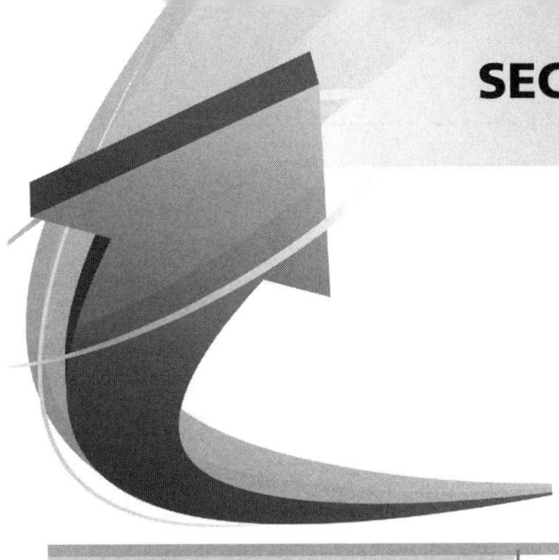

CASE 1.32
Neisseria gonorrhea | Level 2

Demographics

PATIENT NAME: Rebecca Collins

AGE: 23

SEX: Female

HEIGHT: 5′4″

WEIGHT: 61 kg

RACE: White

ALLERGIES: NKDA

CHIEF COMPLAINT: R. C. is a 23-year-old white female who presents to the urgency care clinic with a chief complaint of increased frequency and dysuria for 3 days. Patient thinks she has a UTI.

HISTORY OF PRESENT ILLNESS: R. C. had no problems with urination until 3 days ago when she had an intense internal burning sensation when going to the bathroom the first thing in the morning. The problem persisted throughout the day with some resolution in pain. That night she had to get out of bed to urinate twice, each time accompanied by dysuria. The following morning she noted the dysuria was accompanied by a mucopurulent discharge, which gradually got worse over the ensuing 2 days, culminating in presentation today. She denies the presence of flank pain, fever, or other accompanying symptoms.

REVIEW OF SYSTEMS: Normal

PAST MEDICAL HISTORY: R.C. reports a history of two UTIs while she was in college, occurring 2 and 4 years ago. She also reports being diagnosed with genital HSV about a year ago. The remainder of her history is unremarkable, with the exception of occasional seasonal allergies, and is noncontributory.

SOCIAL HISTORY: Single, never married, and lives alone; sexually active and currently involved in a monogamous, heterosexual relationship; involved with new partner for around 4 weeks; currently taking oral contraceptives; partner does not use condoms; alcohol use—2 to 3 drinks per month; caffeine use—1 to 2 cups per day; denies tobacco and illicit drug use

FAMILY HISTORY: Father—alive, age 50; mother—alive, age 47; one brother, age 21; one sister, age 19

Vaccine History: Up-to-date

Physical Examination

Gen: Well-nourished, white female in NAD

VS: BP 117/68 mm Hg, HR 65 bpm, RR 18 rpm, T 37.2°C, Ht 5′4″, Wt 61 kg

HEENT: Normal

Lungs: Clear breath sounds

CV: RRR with normal S1/S2 and no audible murmur

Skin: No erythema or petechiae

GU: Mild erythema of external genitalia, moderate cervical erythema with mucopurulent discharge, no lesions

Laboratory and Diagnostic Tests

Hemoglobin: 14.5 g/dL

Hematocrit: 40%

Platelets: 325,000 cells/mm^3

WBC: 7,800 cells/mm^3 with 75% PMNs, 20% lymphocytes, 4% monocytes, 1% eosinophils

Urinalysis: Appearance cloudy, color yellow, ketones negative, specific gravity 1.020, urobilinogen 0.2, blood trace, bilirubin negative, glucose negative, protein negative, pH 6.00, WBC 65 cells/hpf, RBC 5 cells/hpf, bacteria few, nitrite negative, leukocyte esterase negative

Cervical Smear: Gram stain 4 + WBC, 4+ gram-negative diplococci

Diagnosis

Gonorrhea

Medication Record

Multivitamin OTC

Ferrous sulfate OTC

Cetirizine 10 mg po daily

Ortho-Novum 7/7/7 use as directed

SELF-ASSESSMENT QUESTIONS

1. Empiric antimicrobial coverage should include agent(s) that are active against what organism(s)?
2. What is the most appropriate treatment regimen for R. C.'s infection?
3. What are potential complications of untreated gonorrhea?
4. How long should R. C. be counseled to abstain from sexual intercourse?
5. If R. C. has been pregnant and had a history of an anaphylactic reaction to cephalexin, what is the most appropriate agent to empirically treat gonorrhea?
6. If R. C. had presented with complaints of tender joints and arthritic symptoms, what would be the diagnosis and, if needed, what would be the recommended treatment regimen?

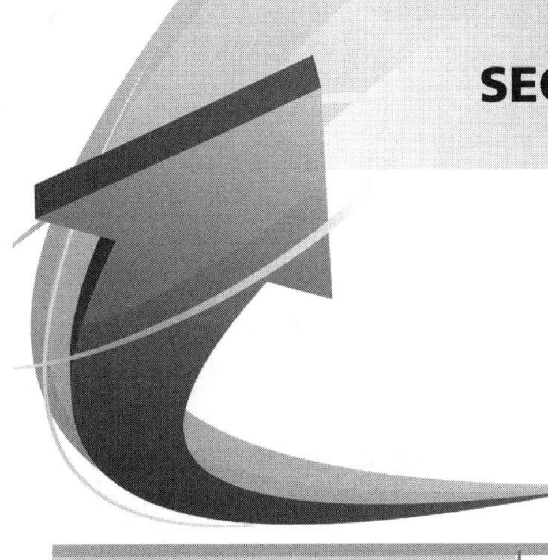

CASE 1.33
Genital Herpes | Level 3

Demographics

Patient Name: Tammy Johnson

Age: 35

Sex: Female

Height: 5′6″

Weight: 60 kg

Race: White

Allergies: NKDA

Chief Complaint: T. J. is a 35-year-old woman who presents to the ambulatory clinic this morning with a complaint of genital pain.

History of Present Illness: T. J. woke up 2 days ago with genital pain. She was concerned that she may have a UTI and started drinking large quantities of fluids. She took two acetaminophen 500 mg every 6 hours for several doses to treat the pain, without relief. Frustrated by the lack of pain resolution with acetaminophen, she presented to the clinic for evaluation. She indicated to the nurse in the clinic on questioning that she has had no symptoms other than the pain.

Review of Systems: Negative except as noted previously

Past Medical History: T. J. was diagnosed with genital herpes 3 years ago. She had two recurrent genital herpes episodes last year and has already had three recurrences during the first 8 months of this year. T. J. typically presents to the clinic with each recurrence for treatment.

Social History: Divorced, lives alone, has no children; dating, has multiple sex partners, partners use condoms; tobacco use—1 pack per day × 20 years; alcohol use— 1 to 2 drinks per day socially on weekends; drug use—denied

Family History: Noncontributory

Vaccine Record: Childhood and adolescent series completed, including HPV × 3 doses and hepatitis A × 2 doses

Physical Examination

Gen: WDWN female in mild-to-moderate pain

VS: BP 118/78 mm Hg, HR 68 bpm, RR 16 rpm, T 36.8°C, Wt 60 kg

HEENT: PERRLA, oral cavity without ulcers or lesions

Chest: Clear to auscultation and percussion

Abd: Soft, nontender

Neuro: Alert and oriented × 3

GU: Two shallow ulcers noted on labia; no abnormal discharge or vaginal bleeding noted

Laboratory and Diagnostic Tests

Sodium: 141 mEq/L

Potassium: 4.1 mEq/L

Chloride: 101 mEq/L

CO_2 Content: 25 mEq/L

BUN: 16 mg/dL

Serum Creatinine: 0.7 mg/dL

Glucose: 99 mg/dL

AST: 17 units/L

ALT: 24 units/L

ALP: 63 units/L

Bilirubin, Total: 0.4 mg/dL

Bilirubin, Direct: 0.1 mg/dL

Hemoglobin: 14.4 g/dL

Hematocrit: 42.1%

Platelets: 285,000 cells/mm^3

WBC: 7,400 cells/mm^3 with 64% segs, 1% bands, 30% lymphocytes, 5% monocytes

Genital Swab: Culture positive for HSV

Diagnosis

Genital herpes

Medication Record

Acyclovir 400 mg po tid × 5 days, filled three times in last year and a half

SELF-ASSESSMENT QUESTIONS

1. What is an appropriate treatment regimen that could be effectively used to treat T. J.'s acute genital HSV episode?
2. The primary goal of treatment of recurrent episodes of HSV with acyclovir is which of the following?
   a. Eradication of HSV through cidal effects on the virus
   b. Symptomatic control through inhibition of viral replication
   c. Concomitant prevention of herpes zoster infections
   d. Management of bacterial superinfection caused by virus-induced tissue damage
   e. Prevent acquisition of sexually transmitted diseases other than HSV from an infected partner
3. What therapy should be recommended for chronic suppressive therapy if T. J. began to experience greater than 10 episodes per year of genital HSV?
4. Had T. J. been diagnosed HIV positive with severe, disseminated HSV infection, what would be the most appropriate treatment regimen to use?
5. Which of the following counseling points is appropriate for T. J.?
   a. Episodic therapy reduces the risk of transmission.
   b. Sexual transmission occurs only during symptomatic periods.
   c. Her sex partner(s) should not worry about being infected unless the partner(s) has/have symptoms.
   d. It is not necessary for T. J. to inform current and future sex partners that she has genital herpes.
   e. T. J. should abstain from sexual activity with uninfected partners when lesions or prodromal symptoms are present.
6. T. J. becomes pregnant and has two recurrent episodes during pregnancy. The infant is born, and the pediatrician is concerned for disseminated neonatal herpes. What is the appropriate treatment regimen for the infant?

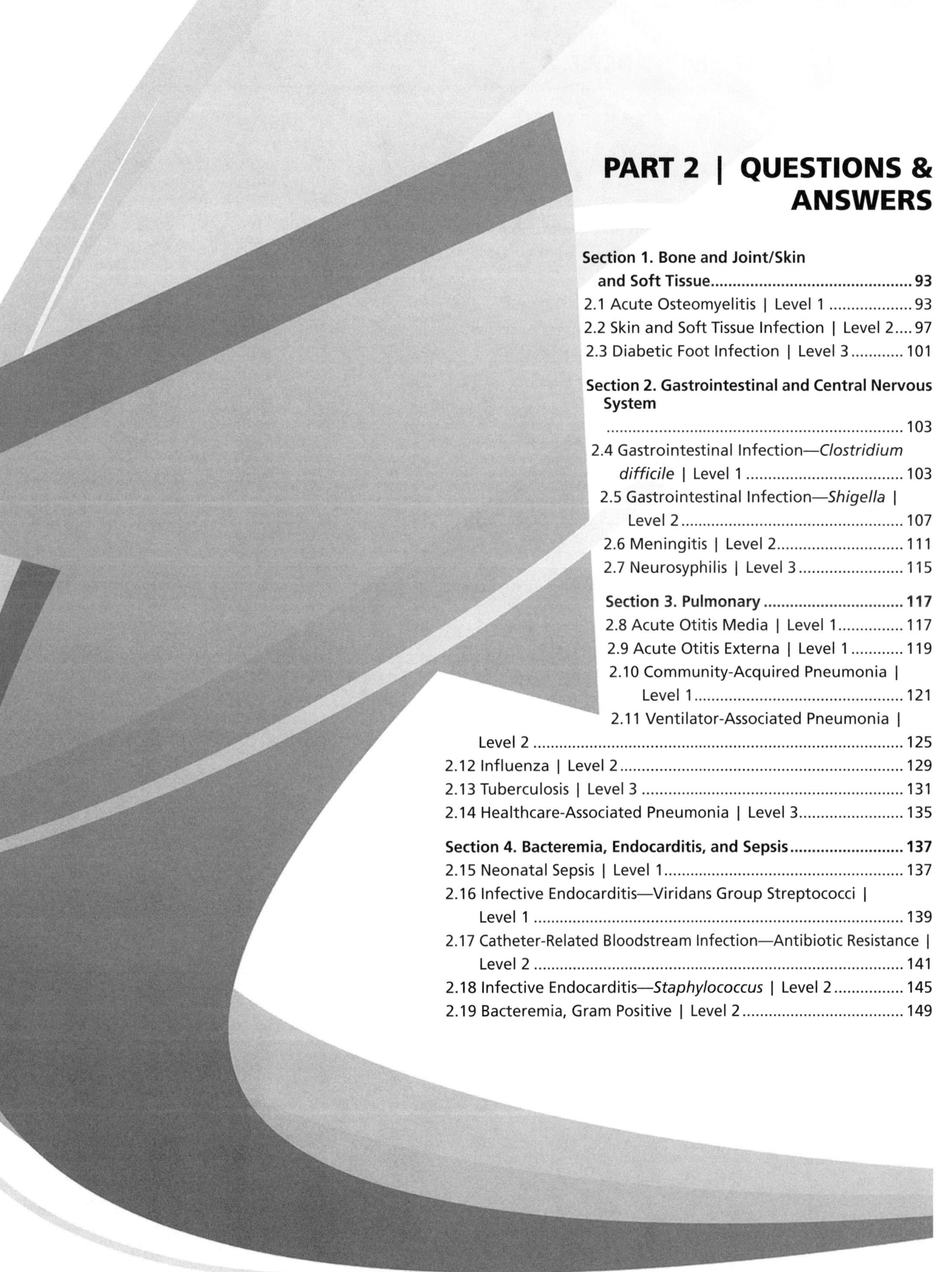

PART 2 | QUESTIONS & ANSWERS

PART 2 | QUESTIONS & ANSWERS

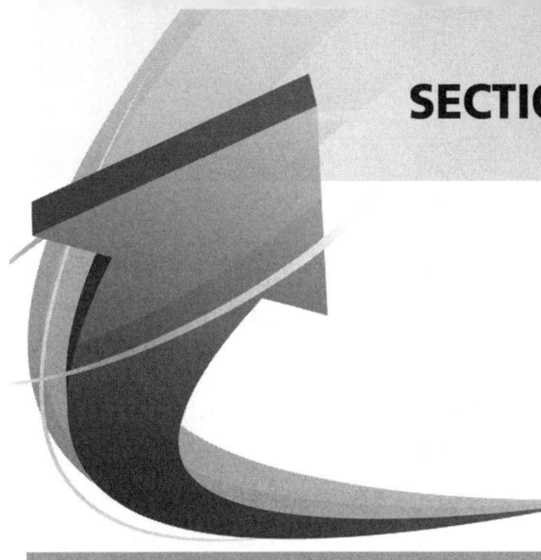

CASE 2.1
Acute Osteomyelitis | Level 1

SELF-ASSESSMENT ANSWERS

1. **What are the clinical findings of osteomyelitis and what are potential complications of the disease?**

   Elevated temperature and WBC count are indicative of acute infectious processes and could be expected to be elevated as in this case. Although relatively nonspecific, the increased ESR and CRP indicate inflammation and are consistent with osteomyelitis. Blood cultures may be positive in patients with acute osteomyelitis, particularly with hematogenous-spread osteomyelitis. Although not very sensitive, the blurred margins presented on the x-ray can be an early sign of osteomyelitis. Finally, the HR and RR of the patient are not elevated significantly, but when considering the physical condition of the patient, these modest compensatory elevations could be a result of an infectious process.

   Necrotic bone, sepsis, chronic infections, bone deformities, and required amputation are all possible sequelae from osteomyelitis. In some cases, infection within bones can spread into a nearby joint causing septic arthritis.

2. **What is the most likely microbiologic etiology for the suspected osteomyelitis?**

   The most appropriate choice is *S. aureus*, given the time to presentation postsurgery. The source is most likely skin contamination via surgical wound. Other organisms that could cause osteomyelitis in adults and children include *Staphylococcus epidermis*, *P. aeruginosa*, *E. coli*, *Streptococcus pyogenes*, and *Streptococcus pneumoniae*. *S. epidermis* is more likely a causative organism when foreign materials are present, such as a metal plate. *Salmonella* species are a common cause in patients with sickle cell disease. *Kingella kingae* should also be considered as a source in children younger than 4 years of age.

3. **M. T. appears very agitated and preoccupied on initial presentation to the emergency department. He explains that he has tickets to a sold-out concert for that evening and was hoping to get a "shot of some kind" and then be sent home with oral antibiotics. His classmate was recently prescribed oral ciprofloxacin for a wound infection, and he was hoping to get a similar prescription. Which of the following counseling points**

regarding treatment of his osteomyelitis is *not* correct?

a. Only parenteral antibiotics are used in the management of osteomyelitis.

b. Antibiotics used in the treatment of osteomyelitis generally are given in high doses.

c. Early antibiotic therapy may reduce the need for surgery.

d. Ciprofloxacin has poor activity against staphylococci and would not be a good initial antibiotic choice for him.

e. The duration of antibiotic therapy for osteomyelitis is usually 4 to 6 weeks.

Answer a is correct. Antibiotics used in the management of acute osteomyelitis should be given in high doses, and, at least initially, are generally given intravenously (b). However, patients may be switched later to oral antibiotics to complete therapy if they have a clinical response to parenteral antibiotics, if there is an appropriate oral agent available, and if medication adherence can be ensured. Early antibiotic therapy may reduce the need for surgery because a delay in treatment may allow the development of bone necrosis, thus making it more difficult to eradicate the infection (c). Ciprofloxacin has inadequate activity against *S. aureus*, and there is some concern regarding staphylococci resistance to fluoroquinolones (d). The duration of treatment for osteomyelitis is typically 4 to 6 weeks, with failure rates occurring in shorter antibiotic regimens (e). Longer durations of treatment may be warranted. Therefore, answer a is the correct answer because both parenteral and oral antibiotics are used for treating osteomyelitis.

4. M. T. is initiated on vancomycin but does not tolerate it, so the physician decides to change to a different parenteral antibiotic regimen. After consulting with the pharmacist, either linezolid or daptomycin is recommended as an alternative option. Which one of the following statements is *not* correct regarding IV linezolid and daptomycin therapies?

a. Selective serotonin reuptake inhibitors (SSRIs), such as fluoxetine, may cause a serotonin syndrome when administered with linezolid.

b. Thrombocytopenia is a recognized adverse effect of linezolid.

c. Concurrent ingestion of large amounts of tyramine-containing foods, such as aged or matured cheese, with daptomycin may cause sudden and severe high blood pressure.

d. Creatine kinase concentrations should be monitored at least weekly during daptomycin therapy.

e. Concurrent administration of HMG-CoA reductase inhibitors with daptomycin may increase the risk of myopathies.

Answer c is correct. Linezolid has mild monoamine oxidase (MAO) inhibitor properties and interacts with serotonergic agents, such as fluoxetine, so patients should be monitored closely for signs and symptoms of serotonin syndrome with concomitant use (a). Due to its mild MAO inhibitor properties, patients should avoid concurrent ingestion of large amounts of tyramine-containing foods with linezolid (not daptomycin) because this may also cause a serotonin syndrome, including a hypertensive crisis (c). Myelosuppression, namely thrombocytopenia, has been reported with linezolid therapy (b). Tedizolid is another oxazolidnone antibiotic with similar adverse reactions as linezolid. Patients on daptomycin should be monitored for myalgias, and this risk increases when daptomycin is administered with HMG-CoA reductase inhibitors (statins). Creatine kinase concentrations should be checked at least weekly throughout daptomycin therapy, with more frequent monitoring in patients taking statins (d, e). Therefore, the correct answer is c because the adverse effects associated with the mild MAO inhibitor properties are seen with linezolid, not daptomycin.

Of note, it is important for the pharmacist to clarify with the physician, nurse, and/or patient what is meant by the patient "not tolerating" vancomycin prior to changing therapies. Drug infusion reactions, adverse reactions, and true allergic reactions should be differentiated to determine if the patient should or should not receive vancomycin now and in the future.

5. **After receiving 7 days of parenteral antibiotics, the physician decides to switch M. T. to oral therapy. His strain of methicillin-resistant *Staphylococcus aureus* (MRSA) is sensitive to all the expected antibiotics. Which are the options for treating his infection?**

Linezolid, tedizolid, clindamycin, trimethoprim/sulfamethoxazole, minocycline, and doxycycline are all available in both oral and IV formulations. In particular, linezolid's oral tablets approach 100% bioavailability. Daptomycin is available only in a parenteral formulation and does not offer an oral alternative to complete therapy. Telavancin, dalbavain, and oritavancin are also available only in an IV formulation. Tigecycline, although indicated for MRSA infections, is not included in guidelines nor recommended for use due to safety warnings related to an increase in mortality among patients treated with tigecycline compared to other antibiotics. Rifampin may also be reported in microbiology reports but should be only used in combination for therapy. It should never be used alone.

6. **Approximately 2 weeks after switching to oral therapy (3 weeks total of oral and parenteral antibiotics), the patient visits you and states a desire to discontinue his antibiotic. He explains that at his last doctor's appointment 2 days ago, the physician told him that he had no fever, his WBC count was back to normal, and the physical exam was unremarkable with no swelling, redness, or tenderness at the surgical wound site. How would you counsel this patient?**

Two weeks of oral therapy (3 weeks total of oral and parenteral antibiotics) is not sufficient time for treatment of osteomyelitis. It is advised that 4 to 6 weeks of adequate antibiotic therapy be administered. In addition, high doses of antibiotics are used in treating osteomyelitis. Patients may be able to complete their course of therapy with oral antibiotics if signs of active infection have resolved, symptoms have improved, a suitable oral agent is available, and compliance is ensured. More data exist in children versus adults for the success of 4-week therapy versus 6-week therapy. The Infectious Diseases Society of America (IDSA) guidelines recommend that osteomyelitis caused by MRSA be treated a minimum of 8 weeks. Chronic infections may result in an additional 1 to 3 months of therapy.

BIBLIOGRAPHY

Liu C, Bayer A, Cosgrove SE, et al. Clinical practice guidelines by the Infectious Diseases Society of America for the treatment of methicillin-resistant *Staphylococcus aureus* infections in adults and children. *Clin Infect Dis.* 2011;52(3):e18-55.

Moenster RP, Linneman TW, Call WB, et al. The potential role of newer gram-positive antibiotics in the setting of osteomyelitis of adults. *J Clin Pharm Ther.* 2013;38(2):89-96.

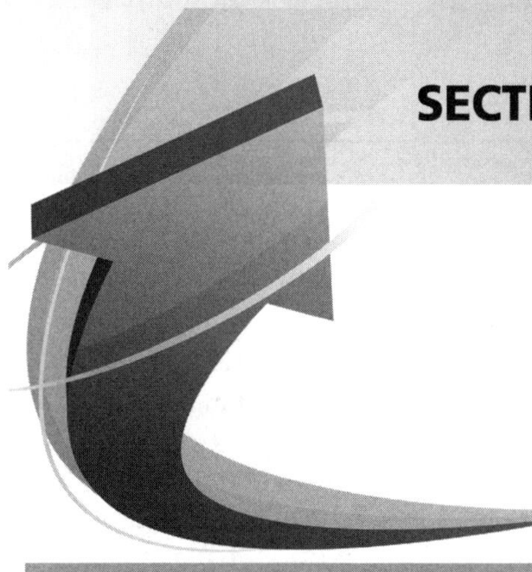

CASE 2.2
Skin and Soft Tissue Infection | Level 2

SELF-ASSESSMENT ANSWERS

1. Name the organisms that are a common cause for the following:

a. Uncomplicated nonpurulent cellulitis

b. Skin infections involving furuncles, carbuncles, or abscesses

a. Although a variety of organisms occasionally cause cellulitis, *Streptococcus pyogenes* is the most common cause of uncomplicated nonpurulent cellulitis. Other organisms that should be on the differential include group C and G streptococci, particularly in diabetics, and *Haemophilus influenzae* in children. Group B strep infections can be seen in newborns. Infections caused by *Staphylococcus aureus* are usually associated with purulent drainage and abscesses. If water exposure occurred, organisms to consider include *Aeromonas* and/or *Vibrio*. *Aeromonas* is common in fresh water, and *Vibrio* is common in salt water. *Clostridium perfringens* can be found infrequently in cellulitis infections; gram-negative organisms such as *Pseudomonas* are not commonly the cause of such infections except in specific patient populations. *Streptococcus pneumoniae* is not associated with skin infections but is the most frequently identified organism in community-acquired pneumonia.

b. Skin infections associated with carbuncles, furuncles, and abscesses are generally caused by *S. aureus*. Furuncles are usually infected hair follicles that develop into a small abscess, whereas carbuncles are a group of furuncles that form an abscess. Infections caused by *S. aureus* generally are associated with abscesses or purulent drainage. Moist heat for small infections and incision and drainage are the treatment of choice for larger infections. Antibiotics are indicated if the patient has systemic signs of infection or extensive cellulitis surrounding the wound. Cellulitis that is diffuse in presentation or does not appear to have an established portal of entry is generally caused by *Streptococcus* species.

2. What are the risk factors for methicillin-resistant *S. aureus* (MRSA) infections, and which oral antibiotics can be used to treat community-acquired MRSA (CA-MRSA) skin infections as an outpatient?

Prior to the late 1990s, virtually all infections associated with MRSA were healthcare related. In the 2000s, widespread cases of CA-MRSA were reported. Infections caused by CA-MRSA usually involve superficial skin infections like boils or furuncles, but more complicated infections can occur. Risk factors for infections caused by CA-MRSA are different than healthcare-related MRSA. Common CA-MRSA risk factors include age (common in pediatrics), steam baths, close skin contact such as participation in contact sports, crowded living conditions such as prisons or military barracks, or poor hygiene. Unlike healthcare-acquired MRSA, CA-MRSA generally remains susceptible to most non-beta-lactam antibiotics. Minocycline and trimethoprim/sulfamethoxazole generally retain activity against CA-MRSA and have been used successfully to treat skin infections caused by CA-MRSA as an outpatient. Oral vancomycin is not absorbed from the gastrointestinal tract and must be administered intravenously. Oral vancomycin should be used only to treat infections in the gastrointestinal tract such as *Clostridium difficile*-associated diarrhea. Although clindamycin can be used to treat CA-MRSA infections, an inducible mechanism of resistance has been reported. Occasionally, therapeutic failures are encountered. Microbiology labs test for inducible clindamycin resistance and report such isolates as resistant. However, if clindamycin is to be used empirically to treat presumed CA-MRSA infections, confirmation of clindamycin sensitivity and appropriate follow-up may be warranted. Oral linezolid is an option for outpatient treatment of MRSA infections, although the cost of twice-daily dosing may be a limiting factor. Tedizolid is a once-daily oxazolidinone approved for MRSA infections as well and is available in an oral formulation.

3. D. H. was placed on vancomycin intravenously for his CA-MRSA. The pharmacist is responsible for adjusting the dose based on levels. After four doses at 1,000 mg IV every 12 hours, his serum trough vancomycin level is 4.5 mg/dL. What should the pharmacist do regarding his vancomycin dose and regimen?

The goal trough vancomycin concentration for skin and soft tissue infections is at least 10 but less than 20 mg/dL. Patients that have osteomyelitis, pneumonia, or meningitis have goal trough concentrations of 15 to 20 mg/dL. D. H. is receiving approximately 13 mg/kg of vancomycin, which is within the normal dosing range of 10 to 15 mg/kg per dose. The dose should not be decreased; his current trough level is below goal. A 50% increase in dose to 1,500 mg every 12 hours should result in a 50% increase in trough, which will not be sufficient to achieve adequate troughs. Decreasing the interval to every 8 hours will result in increased trough concentrations and is a better option than just increasing the dose. More aggressive dosing, such as increasing the dose *and* decreasing the interval, would also be a reasonable action (e.g., 1,250 mg IV q 8 hr) because this patient was septic upon presentation.

4. What if the susceptibility test showed the vancomycin MIC returned as 2 mcg/mL? What should the pharmacist do regarding his vancomycin dose and regimen?

If the vancomycin MIC had returned as 2 mcg/mL, consider changing to another antimicrobial to treat the MRSA infection because of the potential high risk for treatment failure (clinical and bacteriological) with MICs of 2. However, it is important to consider the patient's response (e.g., clinical signs and symptoms, laboratory values, etc.) on current therapy before making a decision to change antimicrobials. Other antimicrobial options could include linezolid, daptomycin, ceftaroline, tedizolid, or trimethoprim/sulfamethoxazole. Telavancin, dalbavancin, and oritavancin are newer lipoglycopeptide antibiotics approved for skin and soft tissue infections. They are available only for the IV route. Clindamycin could be an option, but some clinicians are hesitant to use it for severe MRSA infections due to its characteristics of a bacteriostatic agent and association with inducible resistance. Tigecycline is considered an alternate for MRSA skin and skin structure infections due to an increase in mortality.

5. **In the hospital, D. H. is placed in contact isolation due to his MRSA infection in an attempt to prevent other patients from becoming infected. What infection control procedures are necessary while D. H. is in the hospital?**

MRSA is considered to be a resistant pathogen, and most healthcare facilities have infection control policies that direct preventative measures to decrease patient-to-patient transmission. *S. aureus,* including MRSA, generally colonizes a host's nares prior to causing infection. The primary mode of transmission of MRSA in hospital environments is via healthcare workers' hands. This can occur when a healthcare worker touches an infected patient or comes into contact with contaminated environmental surfaces. The healthcare worker then spreads the bacteria to other patients if preventative measures are not taken. When patients are known to be infected or colonized with MRSA, they should be admitted to a single room or share a room with another MRSA-positive patient. It is not necessary to wear a facemask or protective glasses when treating a person with MRSA, unless the patient has a respiratory infection or the provider may be subject to splashing of infected body fluids. All healthcare workers should wash their hands with soap and water or alcohol-based foam prior to and after coming into contact with each patient, including D. H. The patient should be placed in a private room, and visitors should wear a gown and gloves when touching the patient or the proximal environment. Providing dedicated noncritical patient care medical equipment (used for only that patient) has been shown to be beneficial in preventing the transmission of organisms from patient to patient.

6. **In which of the following skin infections is topical antibiotic therapy most appropriate?**

   a. **Cellulitis in a healthy adult female**
   b. **Impetigo in a teenager**
   c. **Erysipelas with associated fever and chills**
   d. **Deep bite wound received by a human**
   e. **Diabetic foot infection**

Answer b is correct. Cellulitis involves infection of the dermis (a), whereas impetigo involves infection of the epidermis. The former generally involves treatment with systemic antibiotics, whereas the latter generally can be treated with topical antimicrobials such as mupirocin or retapamulin. Impetigo can also successfully be treated with oral antibiotics (b). Human bite wounds and diabetic foot infections are infections that generally require systemic antibiotic therapy along with debridement and source control (d, e). Erysipelas is related to cellulitis (more superficial) (c) and is also usually treated with systemic antibiotics when other systemic symptoms are present (such as fever and chills).

7. **What if D. H. presents to the ED with only a cut on the bottom of his foot that looks infected? He has fever, chills, and an elevated WBC count. He states that 2 days ago he stepped on a piece of broken glass at the bottom of a swimming pool and that the glass cut his foot. The physician wants to prescribe cephalexin as empiric treatment for this skin and soft tissue infection. What should the pharmacist say?**

   a. **Infections that occur in under-chlorinated swimming pools or hot tubs can be caused by *Pseudomonas aeruginosa*. Cephalexin does not possess activity against *P. aeruginosa*, and the patient should receive oral ciprofloxacin.**
   b. **Infections that occur in under-chlorinated swimming pools or hot tubs can be caused by *P. aeruginosa*, which has high intrinsic resistance to all oral cephalosporins, and moxifloxacin should be used to treat the infection.**
   c. **This foot infection is likely caused by a food and water contaminant like *Shigella* or *Salmonella* and should be treated with oral trimethoprim/sulfamethoxazole.**
   d. **This foot infection is likely caused by *Streptococcus pyogenes*, a common cause of cellulitis. Cephalexin is an**

excellent choice, and I will fill the prescription right away.

e. **Ertapenem should be prescribed rather than cephalexin to cover for likely pathogens including *P. aeruginosa*.**

Answer a is correct. Puncture wounds received while in an under-chlorinated swimming pool or hot tub can result in *P. aeruginosa* infection. *Pseudomonas* is highly resistant to many antibiotics and should be treated with an antipseudomonal fluoroquinolone (ciprofloxacin or levofloxacin) (a), IV piperacillin, piperacillin/tazobactam, IV ceftazidime, or IV cefepime. The newer fluoroquinolones (moxifloxacin and gemifloxacin) do not provide reliable *P. aeruginosa* coverage (b). Although trimethoprim/sulfamethoxazole has activity against *Shigella* or *Salmonella*, which are gram-negative bacteria, it does not possess activity against *P. aeruginosa* (c) and cellulitis because these organisms are rare. Wounds of this kind can also cause deep tissue abscess, fever, and leukocytosis. If possible, a culture should be obtained and treatment should continue for at least 2 weeks. Cephalexin would provide coverage against *S. pyogenes*, but because of the risk for *Pseudomonas* it is not an optimal treatment (a, d). Ertapenem does not cover *P. aeruginosa* (e).

BIBLIOGRAPHY

Liu C, Bayer A, Cosgrove SE, et al. Clinical practice guidelines by the Infectious Diseases Society of America for the treatment of methicillin-resistant *Staphylococcus aureus* infections in adults and children. *Clin Infect Dis*. 2011;52(3):e18-55.

Singer AJ, Talan DA. Management of skin abscesses in the era of methicillin-resistant *Staphylococcus aureus*. *N Engl J Med*. 2014;370(11):1039-47.

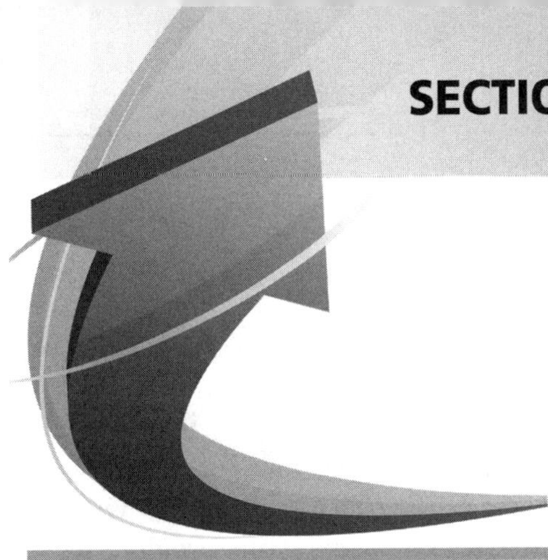

CASE 2.3
Diabetic Foot Infection | Level 3

SELF-ASSESSMENT ANSWERS

1. What is the most likely microbiologic etiology for a diabetic foot infection?

Mild diabetic foot infections are generally monomicrobial. Severe diabetic foot infections are usually polymicrobial with gram-positive and gram-negatives aerobes and anaerobes. Gram-positive cocci (*Staphylococcus* and *Streptococcus*) and Enterobacteriaceae are typically identified. *Pseudomonas* can be seen in more severe infections and usually in patients who live in warm environments or frequently are in the water. Anaerobic organisms are usually seen in infections with necrotic or foul-smelling wounds or ischemia.

2. Based on the *2012 Infectious Diseases Society of America Clinical Practice Guideline for the Diagnosis and Treatment of Diabetic Foot Infections*, what is the classification of this diabetic foot infection?

Based on the IDSA guideline's infection severity rating, this diabetic foot infection would be classified as severe because the patient meets criteria for a local infection (erythema, swelling, warmth, and discharge) and has two signs of systemic inflammatory response syndrome (elevated temperature and increased WBC count).

3. Develop an empiric treatment plan for J. T.

Because J. T.'s infection is classified as severe, he should be hospitalized and receive empiric IV therapy followed by oral therapy for 2 to 4 weeks. Antimicrobial therapy should cover gram-positive, gram-negative (including *Pseudomonas* as he frequents the water several times weekly), and anaerobic organisms. Initial therapy could include daptomycin, linezolid or vancomycin plus aztreonam, cefepime, ceftazidime, imipenem/cilastatin, or piperacillin/tazobactam. If aztreonam, cefepime, or ceftazidime is selected, additional anaerobic coverage should be considered. An optimal therapy has not been determined. Debridement should occur of the wound as well as appropriate wound care. Ceftaroline is an antibiotic that covers the pathogens for severe diabetic foot infection, but it has yet to be studied in this population. Several other newer antibiotics have been approved for skin and skin structure infections, but clinical trials have excluded patients with diabetic foot infection.

4. **J. T.'s blood cultures report no growth, and his wound cultures report positive for *Pseudomonas aeruginosa* and *Bacteroides fragilis*. Susceptibilities are listed below:**

<u>*P. aeruginosa*</u>

Cefepime	I
Ciprofloxacin	R
Gentamicin	S
Imipenem/cilastatin	S
Piperacillin/tazobactam	S
Tobramycin	S

<u>*B. fragilis*:</u> No susceptibility report provided

What alterations, if any, would you recommend for your treatment plan?

If you had initiated an antibiotic that reported back as resistant or intermediate, it would be best to change to an antibiotic for which this pseudomonal isolate has susceptibility. Because MRSA is not reported, coverage for this pathogen is not needed. Likely, select an antibiotic that will cover both organisms and de-escalate treatment to piperacillin/tazobactam.

5. **You are asked to be the pharmacist member on a new antimicrobial stewardship team. The team is deciding how to measure adult antibiotic use in the inpatient setting. What do you suggest the team uses for metrics?**

Antimicrobial stewardship teams are focused to improve the quality of antibiotic prescribing thus improving clinical outcomes and reducing healthcare costs. Numerous measures could be used for outcomes and benchmarking. These include defined daily dose (DDD)/1,000 patient days, days of therapy (DOT)/1,000 patient days, days of therapy/1,000 admissions, length of therapy/discharge or admissions, length of therapy/1,000 patient days, days of therapy/length of therapy ratio, or proportion of patients receiving antibiotic therapy. Any of these would be an appropriate metric for stewardship, but the most common metrics are DDD and DOT. Currently, the most common metric in institutions in the United States is DOT/1,000 patient days. This data report could be used internally to identify where to focus resources to decrease antibiotic use as well as used for comparisons to benchmark against other institutions. Other outcomes measurable by an antimicrobial stewardship team include reduction in antimicrobial resistance and reduced adverse drug events.

6. **What if J. T. had presented with a mild diabetic foot infection and the wound culture grew MRSA? What would be the treatment regimen and duration?**

If the infection had been classified as mild and MRSA was suspected or known, J. T. could have received doxycycline 100 mg orally every 12 hours for 1 to 2 weeks. If the infection was slow to heal, the treatment duration could be extended to 4 weeks. Other oral MRSA treatment options include clindamycin, minocycline, or linezolid. Because J. T. has an allergy to sulfa (hives), it would be best to avoid sulfamethoxazole/trimethoprim. Otherwise, it would be an option for MRSA infections.

BIBLIOGRAPHY

Dellit TH, Pwens RC, McGowen JE, et al. Infectious Diseases Society of America and the Society for Healthcare Epidemiology of America guidelines for developing an institutional program to enhance antimicrobial stewardship. *Clin Infect Dis.* 2007;44(2):159-77.

Ibrahim OM, Polk RE. Antimicrobial use metrics and benchmarking to improve stewardship outcomes: methodology, opportunities, and challenges. *Infect Dis Clin North Am.* 2014;28(2):195-214.

Lipsky BA, Berendt AR, Cornia PB, et al. 2012 Infectious Diseases Society of America clinical practice guideline for the diagnosis and treatment of diabetic foot infections. *Clin Infect Dis.* 2012;54(12):e132-73.

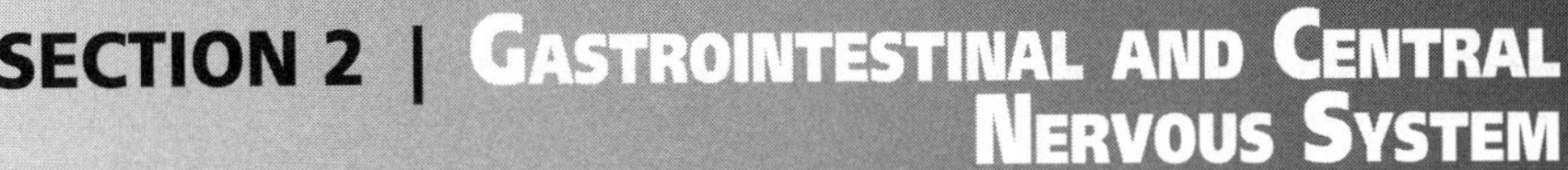

CASE 2.4

Gastrointestinal Infection—*Clostridium difficile* | Level 1

SELF-ASSESSMENT ANSWERS

1. Develop a pharmacologic plan for the treatment of the CDI.

C. difficile is a gram-positive, spore-forming anaerobic bacillus. The treatment of a CDI would include antibiotics such as oral or IV metronidazole, oral vancomycin, or oral fidaxomicin. Because this is J. W.'s first episode of *C. difficile* and he is hemodynamically stable, oral metronidazole 500 mg po three times daily for 10 to 14 days would be an appropriate plan. Metronidazole is the recommended drug of choice for mild-to-moderate infections. Oral vancomycin is warranted for severe infections, and oral vancomycin and IV metronidazole can be used in combination for severe, complicated infections. Fidaxomicin was approved for treatment of CDIs in mid-2011, but current U.S. guidelines lack inclusion of the drug. It was shown to be noninferior to vancomycin for initial cure of a CDI in two Phase III clinical trials. However, institutions generally reserve it for patients who experience multiple recurrent infections or fail metronidazole and/or vancomycin therapy. It is important to note that J. W. should discontinue taking the antiperistaltic agent Imodium because it may obscure symptoms or precipitate complications such as toxic megacolon.

2. Which one of the following statements is *true* regarding *C. difficile* enterocolitis testing and diagnosis?

- **a. *C. difficile* enterocolitis is typically diagnosed in clinical settings by isolation of the organism from the stool.**
- **b. Isolation of the *C. difficile* organism is rare in neonates or infants.**
- **c. False-negative testing results for *C. difficile* are common.**
- **d. The majority of patients in whom the *C. difficile* organism could be isolated will remain asymptomatic for diarrhea.**
- **e. Laboratory testing for *C. difficile* is recommended in all ICU patients because outbreaks commonly occur in this setting.**

Answer d is correct. Although *C. difficile* is not part of the bowel normal flora, it can be isolated in virtually all populations including healthy persons (d). As such, testing of asymptomatic patients and nondiarrheal stools is not recommended. It commonly colonizes neonates and infants with an estimated carriage rate of 30% to 70% (b).

Pathogenic strains cause enterocolitis by secretion of cytotoxins A or B, and the diagnosis is based on isolation of the toxin rather than the organism in most clinical settings (a). Strains that do not produce toxins are nonpathogenic for colitis. Although false-positive testing results (c) are a concern with present testing methodology, a negative testing result can be trusted. Because not all strains of the bacteria are pathogenic for disease and over 50% of patients in whom the organism can be isolated are asymptomatic for diarrhea or evidence of colitis, they can be defined as carriers versus being infected.

3. **Name at least three risk factors for developing a CDI.**

Antimicrobial exposure is a modifiable risk factor for CDIs. Almost all antibiotics have been associated with CDIs. Fluoroquinolones antimicrobials have emerged in the past decade as an important risk factor for CDI, having been associated with NAP1/BI/027 strain that causes severe enterocolitis. Cancer chemotherapy has immunosuppressant and antimicrobial effects, as does the treatment for HIV disease, and both are well-accepted risk factors for the disease. Advanced age has been long known to be an important risk factor for CDI. Duration of hospitalization is also a risk factor. Proton pump inhibitor therapy has been found in several studies to be associated with an increased risk of CDI, and the FDA recently added warnings to this class of acid-suppressing medications. However, a link between CDI and the H_2 blockers has not been established to date. Other risk factors include gastrointestinal surgery or manipulation of the gastrointestinal tract.

4. **Which of the following statements is *true* regarding metronidazole (Flagyl) treatment of *C. difficile* enterocolitis?**

   a. **The drug is effective only if given by the oral route of administration.**
   b. **Relapse rate following a course of metronidazole is less than 2%.**
   c. **The drug is an appropriate first choice in patients of all conditions and ages with *C. difficile* enterocolitis.**
   d. **The failure rate for metronidazole treatment of *C. difficile* enterocolitis appears to be increasing.**
   e. **A 3- to 5-day course of metronidazole therapy may be used in patients presenting with mild *C. difficile* enterocolitis.**

Answer d is correct. Current treatment guidelines recommend metronidazole for the initial treatment of mild-to-moderate disease. Metronidazole can be used in the treatment of *C. difficile* enterocolitis by either the oral or IV route (a). The relapse rate following a course of metronidazole is estimated to be between 10% to 20% (b), and evidence suggests failure rates to metronidazole have been increasing (d). Metronidazole is not recommended for use in all patient populations (c). The drug is not recommended for patients who are pregnant; in these situations, oral vancomycin is preferred. Treatment duration of therapy of 10 to 14 days is recommended in all *C. difficile* patients treated with metronidazole regardless of disease severity; there are insufficient data to support a duration of therapy shorter than 10 days (e).

5. **A medical resident asks you when vancomycin should be used as an appropriate alternative to metronidazole for *C. difficile* enterocolitis. Vancomycin should be considered for therapy in all *except* which one of the following patient types?**

   a. **The patient is intolerant to metronidazole.**
   b. **The patient has failed to respond to an adequate course of metronidazole.**
   c. **The patient has gastrointestinal tract complications and must be treated with IV drug therapy.**
   d. **The patient has severe, life-threatening *C. difficile* enterocolitis.**
   e. **The patient is suffering a second recurrence of *C. difficile* enterocolitis.**

Answer c is correct. Although oral vancomycin is considered equally effective as metronidazole for treatment of *C. difficile* enterocolitis (c), it is regarded as second-line therapy for most initial disease episodes because of concern for the development of vancomycin-resistant enterococci colonization, as well as its increased cost. Unlike metronidazole, vancomycin should not be used by the IV route for treatment of *C. difficile* enterocolitis because adequate drug concentrations are not achieved in the intestinal lumen. Vancomycin is recommended alone or with metronidazole when the patient has severe life-threatening enterocolitis and with recurrences (d, e), based on data that the duration of diarrhea may be shortened. The use of oral vancomycin is appropriate in patients who are intolerant to metronidazole (a). Although the initial CDI episode response rates for metronidazole are typically greater than 90%, and the drug may be utilized for the first disease recurrence, vancomycin is recommended in patients who have their second disease recurrence (b).

6. **Which of the following statements is *true* regarding options for the treatment of *C. difficile* enterocolitis?**

   a. **Treatment with recommended pharmacotherapeutic agents is always required when *C. difficile* enterocolitis is diagnosed.**
   b. **Fidaxomicin is a newer treatment option that is superior in efficacy to vancomycin for treatment of an initial episode of *C. difficile* enterocolitis.**
   c. **Fidaxomicin has been proven to be a cost-effective treatment for all patients with recurrent *C. difficile* enterocolitis.**
   d. **Probiotics have been proven to help prevent *C. difficile* enterocolitis when added to antimicrobial therapy.**
   e. **Combination therapy with oral vancomycin plus IV metronidazole is recommended for initial treatment of severe, complicated *C. difficile* enterocolitis.**

Answer e is correct. The initial action that should be taken in a patient with suspected *C. difficile* enterocolitis is to discontinue the offending antimicrobial agent, and this action alone will result in improvement in approximately 30% of patients (a). Fidaxomicin is a newer treatment option that has been shown to be equally effective but not superior to vancomycin therapy for treatment of initial episodes of *C. difficile* enterocolitis (b). Due to a cost greater than that for either vancomycin or metronidazole, it will not be a cost-effective alternative for most patients with *C. difficile* enterocolitis (c). Probiotics have been used with antimicrobial therapy to prevent *C. difficile* enterocolitis development, but evidence has been conflicting, and they are presently not recommended in guidelines for this purpose (d). Combination therapy with vancomycin plus metronidazole may be used in disease recurrences and is recommended for initial treatment of severe, complicated *C. difficile* enterocolitis (e).

BIBLIOGRAPHY

Cohen SH, Gerding DN, Johnson S, et al. Clinical practice guidelines for *Clostridium difficile* infection in adults: 2010 update by the Society for Healthcare Epidemiology of America (SHEA) and the Infectious Diseases Society of America (IDSA). *Infect Control Hosp Epidemiol.* 2010(5);31:431-55.

Kelly CP, LaMont T. *Clostridium difficile*—more difficult than ever. *N Engl J Med.* 2008;359(18):1932-40.

Louie TJ, Miller MA, Mullane KM, et al. Fidaxomicin versus vancomycin for *Clostridium difficile* infection. *N Engl J Med.* 2011;364(5):422-31.

Schutze GE, Willoughby RE, Committee on Infectious Diseases, American Academy of Pediatrics. *Clostridium difficile* infection in infants and children. *Pediatrics.* 2013 ;131(1):196-200.

CASE 2.5
Gastrointestinal Infection—*Shigella* | Level 2

SELF-ASSESSMENT ANSWERS

1. All *except* which one of the following characteristics helped to distinguish bacterial from viral GE in T. K.?

- **a. Recovery of fecal leukocytes from the stool is common in bacterial GE but rare in viral GE.**
- **b. Bloody diarrhea is common in bacterial GE but rare in viral GE.**
- **c. Travel-related GE can be caused by either bacterial or viral pathogens.**
- **d. Elements of dehydration were present in T. K., and those rarely occur with viral GE.**
- **e. Temperature elevations (fevers) are typically more elevated in bacterial compared to viral GE.**

Answer d is correct. Viral GE due to common causes, including rotaviruses and noroviruses, is typically associated with watery diarrhea and vomiting. Usually, the watery diarrhea is noninflammatory, and no fecal leukocytes are found in the stool (a). Although fevers sometimes occur with viral GE, they are mild in nature. Although some types of bacterial GE, such as that caused by *Vibrio cholerae*, may present with a secretory diarrhea profile common to viral etiologies, the presence of fecal leukocytes, bloody diarrhea (b), and fever (e) is suggestive of a bacterial cause and commonly used to make empiric treatment decisions. Both bacterial and viral causes of GE occur in association with ingestion of contaminated food or water, as may occur during travel (c). For example, norovirus outbreaks have occurred on cruise ships and in school systems. Dehydration is common (d) and a primary treatment issue with either bacterial or viral GE.

2. What is the most common pathogen in acute GE in children less than 10 years of age?

Rotavirus is the most common cause of severe diarrhea in children in the world and remains the most common cause for hospitalization from viral GE in the United States. Infection most commonly occurs in children 6 to 24 months of age, and outbreaks are common. Treatment is supportive. Vaccination for rotavirus is available in the United States and administered at 2, 4, and 6 months of age.

3. What was the most important risk factor for the development of shigellosis in T. K.?

The most important risk factor for T. K. was his travel in an area with poor sanitation. Although tainted food is the most common source in the United States, contaminated water is a typical source. Shigellosis typically affects children younger than T. K., although he is within the age spectrum for the infection. Although summer is the time when most shigellosis is encountered, the infection is uncommon in the absence of a risk created by poor sanitation or an epidemic setting. *Shigella* outbreaks are also associated with crowded living conditions, such as child care centers, nursing homes, and group housing scenarios. Specifically, children under the age of 5 years who are in child care settings are at increased risk of *Shigella* infections.

4. Which antimicrobial agent is preferred in current pediatric guidelines as the treatment of choice of shigellosis?

There are no recent practice guidelines for GE from the Infectious Diseases Society of America (IDSA), but guidelines exist from the American Academy of Pediatrics. Azithromycin is the current drug of choice in children with shigellosis, although reduced organism sensitivity to that agent has been recently reported. Increased resistance to ampicillin has also been seen, and amoxicillin is less effective against *Shigella* due to quick absorption from the gastrointestinal tract. Similarly, *Shigella* resistance to TMP/SMX has also increased. Although quinolones like ciprofloxacin are recommended for use in adult patients, they are usually avoided in children. However, ciprofloxacin is an alternate treatment in children. Ceftriaxone is also an alternative to azithromycin use and preferred over a fluoroquinolone in the pediatric population. Treatment is generally for a duration of 5 days. Although mild infections may not require antibiotics, patients with severe disease, dysentery, or immunocompromising conditions should receive treatment with IV antibiotics.

5. All *except* which one of the following statements are true regarding *Shigella* GE in the entire population?

a. Shigellosis is commonly a self-limited disease that does not require antimicrobial therapy.

b. *Shigella sonnei* is the most common cause of shigellosis in the United States.

c. Shigellosis in the United States most commonly occurs in adult patients.

d. Shigellosis is diagnosed by the isolation of the organism in a stool culture.

e. *Shigella* has no natural reservoir in nature and is passed from person to person.

Answer c is correct. Shigellosis is usually a self-limiting disease, with recovery occurring within a week without antimicrobial therapy (a). However, it is important to note that viral shedding may occur for 1 to 4 weeks after the onset of illness. The most common cause of shigellosis in the United States is *S. sonnei* (b), which has replaced *S. flexneri* as the predominant isolate; *S. dysenteriae* is a common cause in undeveloped countries. *Shigella* has no reservoir in nature (e) and is spread person to person in a fecal–oral transmission pattern. The incidence of shigellosis in young children less than 5 years of age is approximately 10 times that seen in adults (c). Shigellosis is diagnosed by the isolation of the organism in a stool culture (d).

6. What type of medication is not recommended for patients like T. K. who suffer from bloody diarrhea and dehydration in association with shigellosis?

Antidiarrheal agents such as diphenoxylate or loperamide slow intestinal motility. They are not recommended in bacterial GE characterized by bloody diarrhea. There is concern that use of the agent may slow gastrointestinal clearance of the infecting organism and worsen the episode.

BIBLIOGRAPHY

Pickering LK, Baker CJ, Kimberlin DW, et al, eds; American Academy of Pediatrics. *Red Book: 2012 Report of the Committee on Infectious Diseases.* 29th ed. Elk Grove Village, IL: American Academy of Pediatrics; 2012.

Sjölund Karlsson M, Bowen A, Reporter R, et al. Outbreak of infections caused by *Shigella sonnei* with reduced susceptibility to azithromycin in the United States. *Antimicrob Agents Chemother.* 2013;57(3):1559-60.

World Health Organization. Guidelines for the control of shigellosis, including epidemics due to *Shigella dysenteriae* type 1. http://whqlibdoc.who.int/publications/2005/9241592330.pdf. Accessed February 26, 2015.

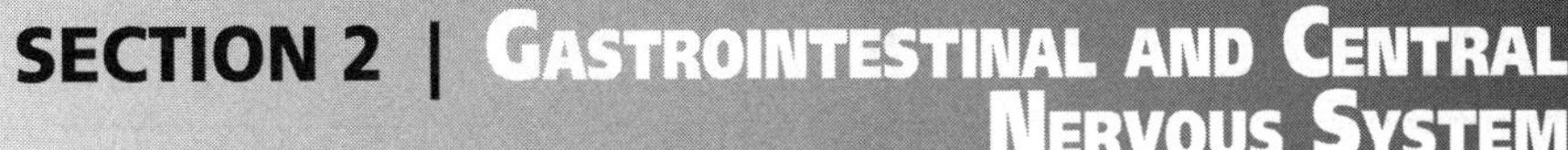

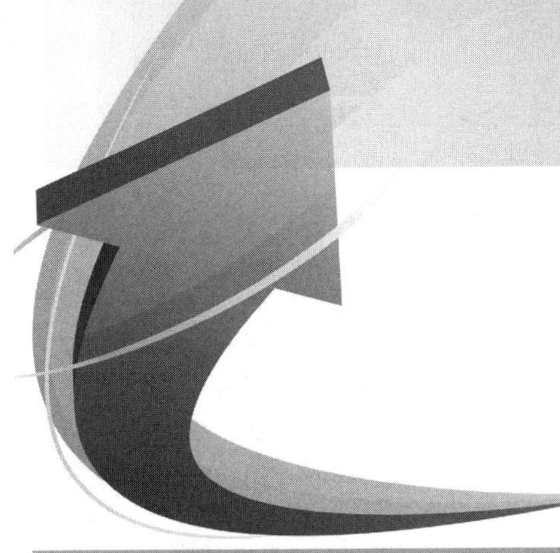

CASE 2.6
Meningitis | Level 2

SELF-ASSESSMENT ANSWERS

1. Name two organisms that are the most likely pathogens in our 22-year-old immunocompetent patient with suspected community-acquired meningitis.

Streptococcus pneumoniae and *N. meningitidis* are the most common causes of traumatic, community-acquired meningitis, with the latter pathogen more likely due to the CSF Gram stain. *Listeria monocytogenes* is an infrequent cause overall, but its frequency is increased in infants younger than 1 month, adults older than 50 years, ethanol abusers, immunocompromised, and patients with comorbid conditions (i.e., diabetes, liver disease, chronic renal disease). *Haemophilus influenzae* type B meningitis was historically the most common cause of meningitis in neonates—but not in adults—and it is no longer of high prevalence in this country due to the widespread use of conjugate vaccines that can now be given as early as 2 months of age. Group B streptococci are common causes of meningitis in the neonate. *Staphylococcus aureus, Acinetobacter baumannii, Pseudomonas aeruginosa,* and *Bacteroides fragilis* are not frequently encountered in community-acquired meningitis but may be encountered in the nosocomial setting, particularly in the patient with CNS trauma (injury or surgery).

2. Which anti-infectives would provide optimal (yet the most narrow spectrum) empiric coverage for meningitis prior to microbiology laboratory findings in this patient?

Ceftriaxone provides effective coverage for *S. pneumoniae* and *N. meningitidis*. Vancomycin is added for coverage of penicillin-resistant isolates of *S. pneumoniae*. Gentamicin, azithromycin, and cefazolin (as well as all other first-generation cephalosporins) poorly penetrate the CNS and should be avoided for treatment of meningitis, although gentamicin may be administered intrathecally when infection is caused by a resistant gram-negative aerobe. Meropenem is an appropriate empiric treatment option for meningitis as well. Daptomycin has not been sufficiently studied clinically at this time, and the pharmacokinetics regarding CNS penetration have not been determined. Metronidazole exhibits a high level of CNS penetration, but activity is limited to anaerobes. As a result, this agent is frequently used when the presence of anaerobic organisms is suspected or confirmed; however, anaerobes are not a frequent cause of community-acquired meningitis. Fluconazole is used exclusively for treatment of fungal infections, which are not common in an immunocompetent individual. Ceftazidime is not required in this patient as *P. aeruginosa* coverage is not necessary. If a patient presenting similar to T. D. had a severe penicillin allergy (i.e., anaphylaxis), the patient should receive chloramphenicol for appropriate coverage against *S. pneumoniae* and *N. meningitidis*. If the penicillin allergy is considered nonsevere (i.e., rash), then it may be necessary to challenge the patient with a cephalosporin because the patient has a relatively safer toxicity profile. In vitro data regarding fluoroquinolone treatment, especially using newer agents, for *N. meningitidis* are positive; clinical data are sparse but emerging.

3. **After 3 days of therapy, the pathogen is determined to be *N. meningitidis*. Which statement most accurately summarizes the utility of corticosteroids in this patient?**

    a. **Dexamethasone should be initiated in this patient because the culture confirmed *N. meningitidis*.**

    b. **Dexamethasone should be initiated in this patient to decrease inflammation associated with concomitant enterovirus infection.**

    c. **Dexamethasone should have been initiated early in this patient, but delay in therapy and uncertain efficacy of dexamethasone in *N. meningitidis* precludes its current utility at this point in the clinical course.**

    d. **Because the culture confirmed *N. meningitidis*, dexamethasone should not be initiated in this patient as it will decrease the penetration of vancomycin, and vancomycin will be unable to treat the *N. meningitidis*.**

    e. **Dexamethasone should not be initiated in this patient due to the patient's leukocytosis. This is a black box warning and an absolute contraindication.**

Answer c is correct. Dexamethasone therapy has been shown to be beneficial in the empiric treatment of certain adult patients' meningitis. The available data suggest that adjunctive dexamethasone should be given prior or concomitant to receiving the first dose of antimicrobial therapy. Patients who have already received antimicrobial therapy are unlikely to benefit from the anti-inflammatory properties of corticosteroids. T. D., however, has not received any corticosteroids at day 3. Therefore, answers a and b cannot be correct. In addition, some experts believe that benefit is only realized in patients with *S. pneumoniae* meningitis. Although dexamethasone has the theoretical ability to decrease vancomycin concentrations in the CSF, clinical data support its use. However, vancomycin is not useful in the treatment of *N. meningitidis*. Therefore, answer d cannot be selected. Finally, the absolute stated in answer e, or the presence of a black box warning, does not exist for dexamethasone and leukocytosis. Therefore, the answer is c. Additional information is available for the reader from the IDSA practice guidelines for the management of bacterial meningitis (available at www.idsociety.org).

4. **What are the prophylaxis regimen options for household contacts of a patient diagnosed with community-acquired meningitis caused by *N. meningitidis*? Does his girlfriend warrant prophylaxis?**

The Advisory Committee on Immunization Practices has published guidelines for the proper prophylaxis of *N. meningitidis* meningitis. These include rifampin 600 mg po every 12 hours × four doses, ciprofloxacin 500 mg po × once, or ceftriaxone 250 mg IM × once (http://www.cdc.gov/mmwr/preview/mmwrhtml/rr5407a1.htm). Chemoprophylaxis is recommended for close contacts of patients diagnosed with *N. meningitidis* meningitis, which includes household contacts, daycare center members, and anyone directly exposed to the patient's oral secretions. Thus, his girlfriend should be provided prophylaxis. Healthcare workers need not receive prophylaxis unless direct exposure to respiratory secretions exists.

5. **T. D. has been in close contact with his sister, who is currently 8 months pregnant, and her physician wants to initiate chemoprophylaxis. Which chemoprophylaxis regimen should she receive?**

Rifampin is an FDA pregnancy category C, and it has been associated with hemorrhagic disease of the newborn. Studies involving pregnant women are generally supportive that rifampin is not a teratogen; however, its use should be avoided if other alternative agents are feasible. Ciprofloxacin is an FDA pregnancy class C drug, due to animal mutagenicity, and alternates should be used when available. Therefore, ceftriaxone 250 mg IM × one dose is recommended, and an FDA pregnancy category class B drug should be used.

6. **Which populations does the Advisory Committee on Immunization Practices (ACIP) currently recommend receiving routine administration of the *N. meningitidis* vaccine?**

Routine administration of the meningococcal conjugate vaccine is recommended by the CDC for preadolescents and young adults (ages 11 to 12) and individuals at increased risk for infection including microbiologists who are routinely exposed to meningococcal bacteria, U.S. military recruits, asplenic individuals, people traveling to countries with meningococcus outbreaks, persons who have terminal complement component deficiencies or human immunodeficiency virus, and those who might have been exposed to meningitis during an outbreak. Infants and children 2 months to 11 years of age and adults, including the elderly, should receive the vaccine if they meet criteria for a high-risk condition. All children should receive a booster dose at 16 years of age.

BIBLIOGRAPHY

Bilukha OO, Rosenstein N; National Center for Infectious Diseases, Centers for Disease Control and Prevention (CDC). Prevention and control of meningococcal disease. Recommendations of the Advisory Committee on Immunization Practices (ACIP). *MMWR Recomm Rep.* 2005;54(RR-7):1-21. http://www.cdc.gov/mmwr/preview/mmwrhtml/rr5407a1.htm. Accessed February 19, 2015.

Centers for Disease Control and Prevention. Immunization Schedules. http://www.cdc.gov/vaccines/schedules/index.html. Accessed February 19, 2015.

Ku LC, Boggess KA, Cohen-Wolkowiez M. Bacterial meningitis in infants. *Clin Perinatol.* 2015;42(1):29-45.

Tunkel AR, Hartman BJ, Kaplan SL, et al. Practice guidelines for the management of bacterial meningitis. *Clin Infect Dis.* 2004;39(9):1267-84 (currently under revision).

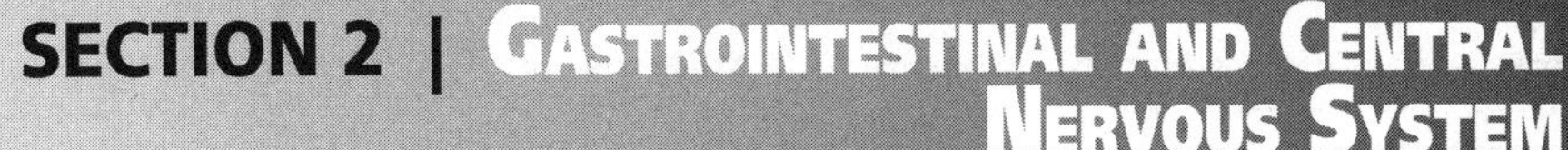

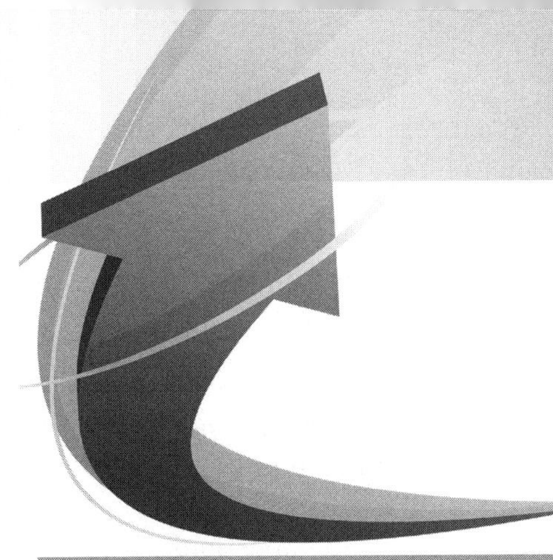

CASE 2.7
Neurosyphilis | Level 3

SELF-ASSESSMENT ANSWERS

1. What is the most appropriate treatment (drug and regimen) for the following:

a. **Neurosyphilis**
b. **Primary syphilis**
c. **Primary syphilis in a penicillin-allergic patient**

a. According to the CDC *Sexually Transmitted Diseases Treatment Guidelines, 2015*, aqueous crystalline penicillin G 18 to 24 million units per day, administered as 3 to 4 million units IV every 4 hours or continuous infusion, for 10 to 14 days remains the drug of choice for treatment of neurosyphilis. A penicillin-allergic patient will require penicillin desensitization.

b. Benzathine penicillin G 2.4 million units IM × 1 is the most appropriate treatment for primary syphilis per CDC *Sexually Transmitted Diseases Treatment Guidelines, 2015*. Infants and children should receive benzathine penicillin G 50,000 units/kg IM, up to the adult dose of 2.4 million units in a single dose. Combinations of benzathine penicillin, procaine penicillin, and oral penicillin preparations are not considered appropriate for the treatment of syphilis as the drug formulation may not penetrate infection sites well.

c. According to the CDC *Sexually Transmitted Diseases Treatment Guidelines, 2015*, doxycycline 100 mg po qid or tetracycline 500 mg po bid for 14 days or azithromycin 2 g po × 1 are alternative treatments for primary syphilis in a patient with a penicillin allergy. Concerns of azithromycin resistance and treatment failures have occurred in several geographical areas of the United States; thus, it should be used with caution and if penicillin or doxycycline is not practical. Ceftriaxone 1 to 2 g daily IM or IV for 10 to 14 days is effective but the optimal dose and duration is questioned.

2. What are characteristic findings of primary, secondary, and tertiary neurosyphilis?

The defining lesion of primary syphilis is the chancre, which forms at the site of inoculation, most commonly the external genitalia. A rash that usually begins on the trunk and proximal extremities and involves the palms of the hands and soles of the feet is a characteristic presentation of secondary syphilis. Other signs of a secondary syphilis infection include mucocutaneous lesions and lymphadenopathy. Cardiovascular or gummatous lesions are characteristic of tertiary syphilis. Meningitis, stroke, cranial nerve dysfunction, or altered mental status are characteristics of neurosyphilis.

3. **G. J. is initiated on treatment and calls the nurse later that afternoon with complaints of fever, headache, and sore muscles. What is the best recommendation for G. J.?**

The Jarisch-Herxheimer reaction occurs shortly after administration of an effective antibiotic—most frequently penicillin—in patients with spirochetal infections. The reaction is thought to be due to pyrogen release after spirochetal lysis. The infection is most frequently associated with initial treatment of syphilis but can occur in patients with other spirochetal infections, including leptospirosis, relapsing fever, and Lyme disease, or bacterial infections, including anthrax, tularemia, brucellosis, and rat-bite fever. The reaction is generally self-limiting, characterized by fever, headache, and myalgias, and is usually treated with NSAID therapy.

4. **What is the drug of choice for the treatment of syphilis in a pregnant patient with a penicillin allergy?**

According to the CDC *Sexually Transmitted Diseases Treatment Guidelines, 2015*, pregnant patients with syphilis should receive parenteral penicillin G for the treatment of syphilis at any stage. If the patient has a penicillin allergy, she should be desensitized.

5. **In monitoring a patient for the treatment of syphilis, what lab change would indicate efficacy of treatment?**

Titers of nontreponemal tests (e.g., RPR) are monitored for efficacy for the treatment of syphilis. A four-fold reduction in RPR is a marker indicating efficacy of treatment. If a patient's titers do not decline four-fold within 6 to 12 months after treatment for primary or secondary syphilis, treatment failure should be considered with additional clinical and serological evaluation. FTA-ABS is a treponemal test that is qualitative only and used to confirm the diagnosis of syphilis.

6. **What combination of labs and clinical disease meets the definition of latent syphilis?**

   a. **(+) RPR, (–) FTA-ABS, (–) clinical disease**
   b. **(+) RPR, (+) FTA-ABS, (+) clinical disease**
   c. **(+) RPR, (+) FTA-ABS, (–) clinical disease**
   d. **(–) RPR, (+) FTA-ABS, (+) clinical disease**
   e. **(+) RPR, (–) FTA-ABS, (+) clinical disease**

Answer c is correct. By definition, latent syphilis is seroreactive without clinical evidence of disease. The RPR is a nontreponemal test and thus a screen. The FTA-ABS is a treponemal test and thus confirmatory for the diagnosis of syphilis.

BIBLIOGRAPHY

Workowski KA, Bolan G; Centers for Disease Control and Prevention (CDC). Sexually transmitted diseases treatment guidelines, 2015. *MMWR Recomm Rep.* 2015;64(RR-03):1-137.

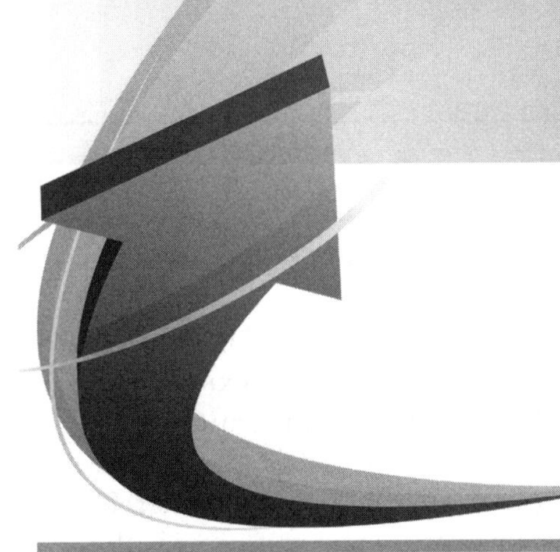

CASE 2.8
Acute Otitis Media | Level 1

SELF-ASSESSMENT ANSWERS

1. Name the most common organisms that cause AOM.

Viruses are the most common pathogens in AOM. Of bacterial causes of AOM, *Streptococcus pneumoniae* currently accounts for approximately 40% of all cases of otitis media. Nontypable *Haemophilus influenzae* accounts for approximately 25% to 30%, and *Moraxella catarrhalis* accounts for about 10% to 15%. Other organisms found in otitis media (~5%) include group A *Streptococcus*, *Staphylococcus aureus*, and anaerobes. Combined viral and bacterial infections are commonly seen in AOM.

2. A resident asks you about the use of TMP/SMX in AOM. How would you respond?

TMP/SMX has a high degree of cross-resistance with penicillin and beta-lactam antibiotics in general. Therefore, if the patient has an infection caused by nonpenicillin-susceptible *S. pneumoniae*, TMP/SMX is most likely an ineffective alternative. It was useful in the past and was often a second-line agent or first-line agent in penicillin-allergic patients. Its use is dramatically lower in pediatrics as safer and more efficacious agents have become available. Not only is cross-resistance a problem, but also the incidence of resistance to TMP/SMX itself is very high and increasing. Most recent studies do not recommend TMP/SMX for treating AOM. Skin reactions have always been a serious complication of sulfa-containing medications. The incidence in children is low, but with many antibiotics that are more efficacious and safer, TMP/SMX should be avoided for AOM. *H. influenzae*, nontypable is the second most common organism causing AOM. At least 10% of the isolates are resistant to TMP/SMX, giving further support to not using TMP/SMX.

3. Describe the mechanism of how *Streptococcus pneumoniae* develops antimicrobial resistance to beta-lactam antimicrobials.

The resistance of *S. pneumoniae* to beta-lactam antimicrobials develops due to alterations in the penicillin-binding protein. By increasing the dose (of amoxicillin, for example) this type of resistance can be overcome. Thus, 90 mg/kg/day of amoxicillin is the appropriate therapeutic dose for otitis media today. The resistance of *S. pneumoniae* to macrolides is due to alterations of the ribosomal binding site and by efflux pumps.

4. Name at least four risk factors for a higher incidence of or increase the risk of developing AOM.

Infants and children exposed to secondhand smoke have a several-fold higher chance of developing AOM and of developing recurrent infections. Day care attendance and anatomic changes such as cleft palate increase the risk of developing AOM. Eustachian tube dysfunction is the most important factor leading to AOM. Numerous etiologies exist for eustachian tube dysfunction; however, when it does not function properly, otitis media and/or sinusitis often develop. Eustachian tube dysfunction prevents removal of inflammatory and infectious material from the middle ear and infection may ensue. Patient age at first occasion of AOM is important. If the infant develops AOM before 6 months of age, the chances of recurring episodes are 50% more likely than in those infants/children whose first episode occurs after 6 months of age. Infants with allergies, atopy, or immunoglobulin G (IgG) deficiencies have a greater risk of developing AOM.

Breastfeeding has been shown to provide protection from developing AOM. Infants who are breastfed until at least 4 months of age have significantly fewer episodes of AOM than children who are bottle-fed. Eliminating pacifier use during the second 6 months of life and avoiding bottle propping can decrease the risk of AOM. Vaccinating the infant with the recommended immunizations is beneficial as well.

5. K. T. returns to her pediatrician 3 days after the initial visit. She is still having fever and is irritable. Her mother was adherent with the antibiotic treatment. The physician feels she failed amoxicillin therapy due to a resistant organism and asks you to develop a therapeutic plan for K. T. What do you suggest?

High-dose amoxicillin therapy (90 mg/kg/day) was appropriate for the initial treatment for AOM because of the increased prevalence of nonpenicillin-susceptible *S. pneumoniae*. This is recommended by the American Academy of Pediatrics for nonpenicillin allergic patients. If the patient has a non-type 1 penicillin allergy, a cephalosporin can be prescribed for AOM, such as cefdinir, cefpodoxime, or cefuroxime. Antibiotics should be changed if the patient is still symptomatic after 48 to 72 hours of antibiotics, and the diagnosis should be re-examined. If a patient fails amoxicillin therapy, amoxicillin/clavulanate is recommended next at a dose of 90 mg/kg/day of amoxicillin with 6.4 mg/kg/day of clavulanate in two divided doses. A 3-day therapy of IM or IV ceftriaxone is an alternative, especially in those not taking oral medications well. If the patient has been initially prescribed amoxicillin/clavulanate or an oral third-generation cephalosporin, IM ceftriaxone for 3 days would be appropriate. TMP/SMX is not recommended for AOM due to a high rate of resistance. Because K. T. has no drug allergies and is tolerating oral medications, amoxicillin/clavulanate should be recommended at a dose of 400 mg po bid × 10 days using the 600 mg/5 mL suspension.

6. What immunizations should K. T. receive at her 1-year-of-age pediatrician visit?

At 1 year of age, K. T. should be administered the *H. influenzae* type B vaccine (Hib), pneumococcal conjugate vaccine (PCV13), inactivated influenza vaccine (IIV), measles, mumps, rubella vaccine (MMR), varicella (chickenpox) vaccine (VAR), and the hepatitis A vaccine (HepA). If she did not already complete her hepatitis B series or receive her third dose of inactivated poliovirus, she would need those as well.

BIBLIOGRAPHY

American Academy of Pediatrics Subcommittee on Management of Acute Otitis Media. Diagnosis and management of acute otitis media. *Pediatrics*. 2004;113(5):1451-65.

Coker TR, Chan LS, Newberry SJ, et al. Diagnosis, microbial epidemiology, and antibiotic treatment of acute otitis media in children: a systematic review. *JAMA*. 2010;304(19):2161-9.

Lieberthal AS, Carroll AE, Chonmaitree T, et al. The diagnosis and management of acute otitis media. *Pediatrics*. 2013;131(3):e964-99.

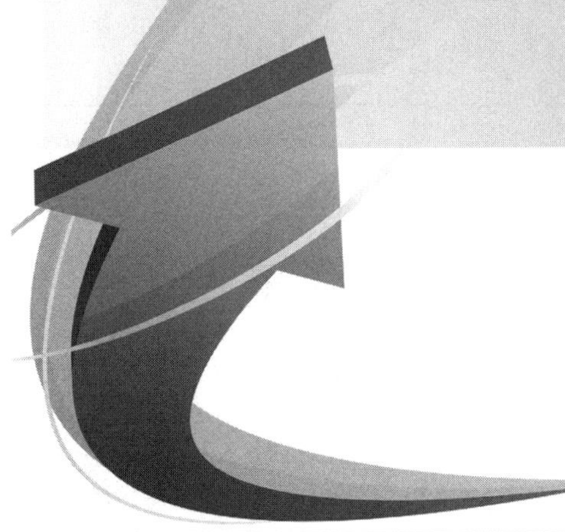

CASE 2.9
Acute Otitis Externa | Level 1

SELF-ASSESSMENT ANSWERS

1. List risk factors and the diagnostic criteria for acute otitis externa.

Excessive cleaning, such as with cotton swabs, or irrigation can injure the ear canal, making it more susceptible to maceration from water trapped by compacted cerumen, inflammation, and infection. Debris from dermatologic conditions and wearing hearing aids may prompt infections. A short ear canal would make it more difficult for water to be trapped, therefore decreasing the risk of acute otitis externa. Acute otitis externa is more commonly seen in warmer climates, increased humidity, or in patients with increased water exposure (swimming, hot tubs, etc.).

The diagnosis of acute otitis externa is made when the following conditions are met: (1) quick onset (within 48 hours) in the past 3 weeks ***and*** (2) symptoms of ear canal inflammation (otalgia, itching, or fullness) with or without hearing loss or jaw pain ***and*** (3) signs of ear canal inflammation (tenderness of tragus, pinna, or both) ***or*** diffuse ear canal edema, erythema, or both with or without otorrhea, regional lymphadenitis, tympanic membrane erythema, or cellulitis of the pinna and adjacent skin.

2. Describe the most common organisms that cause acute otitis externa and develop a general treatment plan for L. R.

The majority (98%) of acute otitis externa in the United States is due to bacteria. The most common pathogens include *Pseudomonas aeruginosa*, *Staphylococcus epidermidis*, and *Staphylococcus aureus*, commonly co-infecting. Infections are usually polymicrobial with additional pathogens being primarily gram-negative organisms. Fungal involvement is rare but could be seen in chronic otitis externa, after treatments of topical antibiotics, or in patients with hearing aids.

Topical antibiotics are the mainstay of treatment for acute otitis externa when no signs of systemic infection are identified (e.g., swelling and pain of the tissues around the mastoid). System antibiotics are rarely indicated. An antiseptic (e.g., acetic acid), antibiotic, corticosteroid, or a combination product may all be considered for initial treatment. Clinical trials have found no significant differences in clinical outcomes of acute otitis externa for various topical combination products (antiseptic versus antimicrobial, quinolone versus nonquinolone antibiotic[s], or steroid antimicrobial versus antimicrobial alone). Cost, adherence, and adverse effects should be considered when selecting a product for a patient. Patients should be assessed for factors that would modify therapy such as nonintact tympanic membrane, tympanostomy tube(s), diabetes, immunocompromised state, and prior radiotherapy.

3. What if L. R.'s tympanic membrane was ruptured? Which of the following is an appropriate otic product that may be used when the tympanic membrane is perforated?

- **a. Ofloxacin otic solution**
- **b. Antipyrine/benzocaine otic solution**
- **c. Ciprofloxacin/hydrocortisone otic solution**
- **d. Neomycin/hydrocortisone/polymyxin B otic solution**
- **e. Acetic acid otic solution**

Answer a is correct. If the tympanic membrane is ruptured or the patient has tympanostomy tubes, nonototoxic formulations must be used. Topical drops that contain alcohol or ototoxic drugs (e.g., aminoglycosides) should be avoided. Ofloxacin otic solution is the only otic solution that is approved for use with a perforated tympanic membrane as quinolone antibiotics are generally safe to use in the middle ear. Antipyrine/benzocaine (b) should be avoided if the tympanic membrane is ruptured. Ciprofloxacin/hydrocortisone (c) is contraindicated because it is nonsterile. Neomycin/hydrocortisone/polymyxin B (d) is contraindicated because it can cause ototoxicity, burning, and stinging. It is specifically contraindicated by the manufacturer for use with a nonintact membrane. Acetic acid solution (e) can cause burning and stinging when used with a perforated tympanic membrane.

4. Describe techniques that a patient should be instructed to do to enhance the contact of an otic solution with the affected area.

First, it is important to appropriately counsel the patient and or caregiver on how to administer topical drops into the ear. Placing a cotton wick in the ear following instillation and manipulating the tragus to effect adequate distribution in the canal are methods that facilitate prolonged contact of the solution with the affected areas of the ear canal and are particularly useful in small children who cannot or will not stay still. An aural toilet can be performed to facilitate the removal of debris from the canal. Warming the solution, usually by holding in hands for 1 to 2 minutes, does not increase the contact of the solution with the affected area but may help minimize dizziness that can occur from instillation of cold drops.

5. The antimicrobial properties of acetic acid, which is a component of some otic preparations, are attributable to its ________.

- **a. Drying properties**
- **b. Hypertonicity**
- **c. Viscosity**
- **d. Acidity**
- **e. Detergent properties**

Answer d is correct. Being a weak acid, acetic acid lowers the pH of the ear canal and creates a local medium that is unfavorable for the growth of organisms.

6. What are common adverse effects of antibiotics found in topical otic preparations?

Topical antibiotics can sensitize the skin, resulting in a dermatitis, which may exacerbate the symptoms of otitis externa and/or interfere with healing. Pruritus is another common adverse effect. Less common adverse effects include discomfort, dizziness, otalgia, vertigo, superinfection, and decreased hearing.

BIBLIOGRAPHY

Rosenfeld RM, Schwartz SR, Cannon CR, et al. Clinical practice guideline: acute otitis externa. *Otolaryngol Head Neck Surg.* 2014;150(1 Suppl):S1-24.

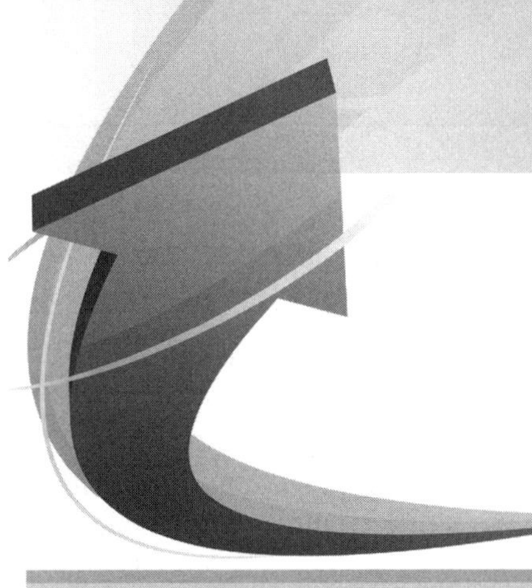

CASE 2.10
Community-Acquired Pneumonia | Level 1

SELF-ASSESSMENT ANSWERS

1. **What are signs and symptoms of community-acquired pneumonia, and what is the most commonly identified pathogen?**

   Fever, increased WBC count with bands, productive cough, and pleuritic chest pain are all findings of pneumonia. The majority of patients presents with fever and cough, but not all patients will have a cough associated with sputum production. Other findings of pneumonia in R. T. include tachycardia, tachypnea, and rales in the left lung. *S. pneumoniae* is the most commonly identified pathogen in community-acquired pneumonia. It is identified in 20% to 60% of all episodes. R. T.'s use of ciprofloxacin 4 weeks ago does not change her diagnosis of community-acquired pneumonia; however, she would not meet criteria for outpatient treatment due to antimicrobial use within the last 3 months per the IDSA guidelines.

2. **All of the following are indicative of an acceptable sputum specimen *except* ________.**

   a. **Greater than or equal to 10 squamous epithelial cells per LPF**
   b. **Greater than 25 PMNs per LPF**
   c. **Less than 10 squamous epithelial cells per LPF**
   d. **Ideally should be collected prior to initiating antibiotic therapy**
   e. **Sputum collection is not required to be performed in all patients based on the 2007 IDSA *Consensus Guidelines on the Management of Community-Acquired Pneumonia in Adults.***

   Answer a is correct. Culturing a poorly collected sputum specimen is a waste of time and money as it will be heavily contaminated with oropharyngeal flora, and the infecting organism will not likely be seen. Therefore, it is important to collect a quality sputum specimen. The IDSA guidelines state that "pretreatment Gram stain/culture of expectorated sputum should be performed only if a good quality specimen can be obtained." Specimen collection should be done prior to beginning antibiotics (d) as the presence of the antibiotic in the specimen may inhibit growth of the organism in culture. However, antibiotics should not be withheld in an emergency situation waiting for a sputum specimen to be collected. Different labs may have varying sputum specimen criteria, but a low number of squamous epithelial cells and a notable presence of PMNs are commonly employed. A quality specimen is often defined as one that contains *less* than 10 squamous epithelial cells and *greater* than 25 PMNs per LPF (a, b, c). The IDSA guidelines also state that sputum samples do not need to be obtained from all patients (e). Table 5 in the 2007 IDSA *Consensus Guidelines on the Management of Community-Acquired Pneumonia in Adults* lists indications in which sputum samples should be obtained. Critically ill patients should have diagnostic testing performed. However, diagnostic testing should not be considered wrong for any patient as these tests have an impact on the care of individual patients. Patients likely to have pathogens, which are not covered by recommended empiric antibiotic regimens, should have the specific pathogens identified to better tailor their antibiotic management. For more information, see *Clin Infect Dis.* 2007;44(supplement 2):S27-72. These guidelines are also found on the IDSA website (www.idsociety.org).

3. R. T. was admitted to the general medical floor of the hospital with a diagnosis of community-acquired pneumonia. Develop an appropriate treatment regimen for R. T. What routine monitoring should be conducted?

Common pathogens for community-acquired pneumonia include *S. pneumoniae, Mycoplasma pneumoniae, Haemophilus influenzae, Chlamydophila pneumoniae, Legionella* species and respiratory viruses such as influenza A and B, adenovirus, respiratory syncytial virus, and parainfluenza. Penicillins, cephalosporins, or respiratory fluoroquinolones are agents with activity against pulmonary gram-positive organisms. Agents with activity against atypical pathogens include macrolides (azithromycin, erythromycin, clarithromycin), doxycycline, and fluoroquinolones. A respiratory fluoroquinolone or a beta-lactam plus a macrolide is appropriate treatment for a nonintensive care unit patient like R. T. Ceftriaxone plus azithromycin is an appropriate regimen for R. T. It will provide coverage for the most common pathogens associated with community-acquired pneumonia. Doxycycline alone is not recommended for hospitalized patients. Levofloxacin plus azithromycin is not appropriate as the regimen is associated with therapeutic duplication. Levofloxacin or moxifloxacin alone are appropriate therapy in a hospitalized patient; however, R. T. recently received ciprofloxacin for treatment of a UTI, and therefore an antibiotic from a different class should be selected to treat R. T.'s pneumonia per the guidelines. Ceftriaxone alone is not appropriate therapy as it will not cover atypical pathogens (*Mycoplasma, Legionella, Chlamydophila*). Therapy guidelines for the management of community-acquired pneumonia are available on the IDSA website (www.idsociety.org).

Patients should be monitored routinely (e.g., on a daily basis) for resolution or improvement in clinical findings, as well as potential adverse effects secondary to antibiotic therapy. Chest x-rays lag behind in improvement (by at least 3 weeks). Chest x-rays should not be routinely used to monitor response to therapy while the patient is receiving antibiotics. However, if the patient fails to demonstrate a clinical response, a follow-up x-ray while on therapy is appropriate. Abnormal findings on chest x-ray clear more slowly than the clinical findings.

4. The microbiology report for R. T.'s sputum culture indicates the pathogen is *Streptococcus pneumoniae* with high-level resistance to penicillin. Which antibiotic would be suitable to treat R. T.?

a. Azithromycin
b. Trimethoprim/sulfamethoxazole
c. Linezolid
d. Doxycycline
e. Cefazolin

Answer c is correct. High-level resistance is indicated by a penicillin MIC of greater than 2.0 mcg/mL. This demonstrates that the pathogen is penicillin-resistant *S. pneumoniae*. These isolates are often referred to as penicillin nonsusceptible *S. pneumoniae*. These organisms should also be considered resistant to first- and second-generation cephalosporins (e), macrolides (a), doxycycline (d), and trimethoprim/sulfamethoxazole (b). Quinolones, clindamycin, vancomycin, telithromycin, linezolid (c), and often third-generation cephalosporins are active against penicillin nonsusceptible *S. pneumoniae*. However, data suggest that in pneumonia, penicillin MICs greater than 4 adversely affect treatment outcome. Therefore, high-dose amoxicillin or ceftriaxone is appropriate, particularly against isolates whose susceptibility is deemed as penicillin-intermediate based on MIC (MIC 0.1 to 1 mcg/mL).

5. List risk factors for penicillin-resistant *S. pneumoniae*.

Risk factors for penicillin-resistant and drug-resistant *S. pneumoniae* include age greater than 65 years, antibiotic therapy within the past 3 months, multiple medical comorbidities, alcoholism, immunosuppression, and exposure to a child in a day care center. Patients with risk factors for drug-resistant *S. pneumoniae* should receive antibiotics that have activity against this pathogen.

6. Which of the following would *not* be recommended as a preventative strategy for community-acquired pneumonia in R. T.?

a. Smoking cessation

b. One dose of Pneumovax® (PPSV23)

c. Intramuscular Fluzone® high-dose (given annually)

d. Intranasal FluMist® (given annually)

e. Proper respiratory hygiene (including hand washing and potentially masks or tissues)

Answer d is correct. Smoking is a risk factor for pneumonia (a). Smoking alters the function of the body's mucociliary transport system. The pneumococcal vaccine is protective against invasive *S. pneumoniae* infection. A single dose of Pneumovax® (PPSV23) is recommended for persons greater than 65 years who have not had it in the previous 5 years (b). The Prevnar 13 vaccine should also be administered to patients 65 years and older who have not received this vaccination. Prevnar 13 should be administered 6 to 12 months prior to PPSV23. The influenza vaccine should be given to those at increased risk of complications, including those 65 years and older. Fluzone® high-dose is an inactivated influenza vaccine recommended in those greater than or equal to 65 years (c). It contains more antigen, which has shown to produce greater antibody levels in the elderly. Whether or not this confers greater immunity has yet to be shown. FluMist® Quadrivalent is an intranasal, live-attenuated influenza vaccine that is recommended only in healthy patients 2 to 49 years old; therefore, R. T. is not eligible for this specific influenza vaccine (d). Proper respiratory hygiene is important in all ages. The CDC website (www.cdc.gov/vaccines) has additional vaccine information and recommendations (e).

BIBLIOGRAPHY

Centers for Disease Control and Prevention. Immunization Schedules. http://www.cdc.gov/vaccines/schedules/index.html. Accessed February 21, 2015.

Mandell LA, Wunderink RG, Anzueto A, et al. Infectious Diseases Society of America/American Thoracic Society consensus guidelines on the management of community-acquired pneumonia in adults. *Clin Infect Dis.* 2007;44(Suppl 2):S27-72.

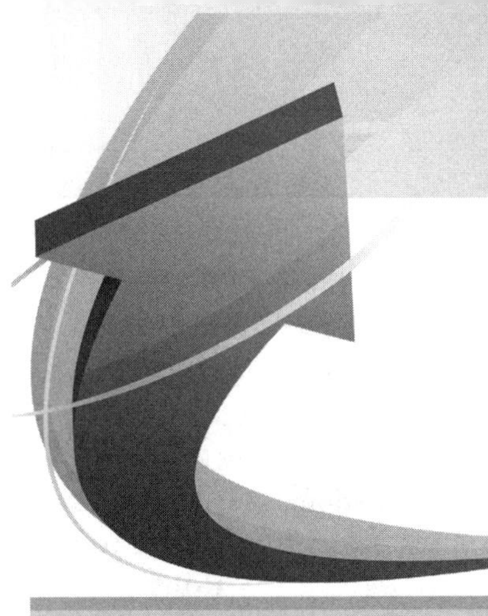

CASE 2.11
Ventilator-Associated Pneumonia | Level 2

SELF-ASSESSMENT ANSWERS

1. **Which one of the following empiric treatment regimens is most appropriate for A. S.?**
   a. **Ceftazidime plus gentamicin plus vancomycin**
   b. **Vancomycin**
   c. **Ceftriaxone**
   d. **Piperacillin/tazobactam plus gentamicin**
   e. **Levofloxacin plus metronidazole**

Answer d is correct. Late-onset nosocomial pneumonias (pneumonias occurring after 5 or more days of hospitalization) are more likely to be caused by gram-negative bacteria (*Pseudomonas* [a], *Enterobacter*, or *Klebsiella*) and *Staphylococcus aureus*. *S. aureus* is not likely as A. S.'s Gram stain demonstrates gram-negative bacilli. A. S. has been intubated and hospitalized for 13 days; therefore, piperacillin/tazobactam plus gentamicin is the most appropriate choice for A. S. (d). He has nosocomial pneumonia; therefore, nosocomial gram-negative pathogens (e.g., *Pseudomonas*, *Enterobacter*, and *Klebsiella*) must be covered. He is currently on ampicillin/sulbactam for his perforated ulcer. Ampicillin/sulbactam does not provide adequate coverage against nosocomial gram-negative pathogens. However, A. S. does need anaerobic coverage for his perforated ulcer; piperacillin/tazobactam will provide this coverage as well. The addition of an aminoglycoside (gentamicin) to piperacillin/tazobactam is usually recommended for the treatment of *Pseudomonas* (d). The combination of an antipseudomonal beta-lactam plus an aminoglycoside provides synergy against *Pseudomonas*. Vancomycin (b) is not appropriate in A. S. because his Gram stain showed gram-negative bacilli. Vancomycin covers only gram-positive organisms. Ceftriaxone does not provide coverage against *Pseudomonas* or anaerobic bacteria. Levofloxacin plus metronidazole (e) is not appropriate therapy for empiric gram-negative coverage for nosocomial pneumonia. A. S. has late-onset nosocomial pneumonia, and the guidelines recommend that empiric therapy for gram-negative coverage include two antibiotics with activity against gram-negative pathogens (must empirically cover for *Pseudomonas*). Quinolones alone are not appropriate empiric therapy for nosocomial pneumonia, especially in a patient in the ICU.

2. **Which one of the following statements is *not* a risk factor for the development of antibiotic resistance?**

    a. **Prior antimicrobial agent use**
    b. **Antimicrobial stewardship**
    c. **Prolonged hospitalization**
    d. **ICU stay**
    e. **Underdosage of antimicrobial agents**

    Answer b is correct. Prior antimicrobial agent use may lead to increasing colonization and potential infection with resistant organisms (a). Prior antimicrobial agent use may have exerted selective pressure, which may have induced resistance as well. Prolonged hospitalization (c) and ICU stays (d) lead to increasing colonization and infection with resistant organisms. Underdosage of antimicrobial agents (e) leads to the emergence of resistant pathogens. Antimicrobial stewardship (b) aims to improve clinical outcomes by minimizing inappropriate use of antimicrobial agents and the emergence of resistant pathogens. For more information on antimicrobial stewardship, see the IDSA website (http://www.idsociety.org/) for antimicrobial stewardship literature. Pharmacists should play a key role in an antimicrobial stewardship program.

3. **The sputum sample grows out *Pseudomonas aeruginosa*. Susceptibilities are as follows:**

Drug	MIC	Breakpoint
Meropenem	0.5	≤ 2
Ceftazidime	4	≤ 8
Ciprofloxacin	2	≤ 1
Piperacillin	4	≤ 16
Gentamicin	1	≤ 4

On the basis of the above culture and susceptibility data, which regimen is now most appropriate for A. S.?

   a. **Piperacillin/tazobactam**
   b. **Ceftazidime plus gentamicin**
   c. **Meropenem plus gentamicin**
   d. **Ciprofloxacin plus gentamicin**
   e. **Ciprofloxacin**

   Answer a is correct. On the basis of culture and susceptibility data, piperacillin/tazobactam (a) is the most appropriate agent based on MIC data and being the most narrow-spectrum agent compared to meropenem. It is the most susceptible agent listed with an MIC of 4 and a breakpoint of 16. The MIC is two dilutions away from the breakpoint, whereas ceftazidime is only one dilution away from the breakpoint; therefore, resistance may emerge. Historically, pseudomonal infections were generally treated with two drugs for synergy purposes. Synergy occurs with a beta-lactam and an aminoglycoside. However, a body of literature supports that you can discontinue the aminoglycoside or other dual therapy agents once susceptibilities are known for the pseudomonal isolate being treated. Overall, the guidelines suggest that monotherapy may be appropriate if the culture does not demonstrate a resistant pathogen. A narrow-spectrum antimicrobial agent would be better than using meropenem (c), a broad-spectrum antibiotic, because sensitivities are known. Ciprofloxacin plus gentamicin (d) is probably the only additive in coverage; however, some believe that the combination is synergistic. Ciprofloxacin (e) with or without gentamicin or ceftazidime plus gentamicin (b) will not provide anaerobic coverage, which is optimal when treating a perforated ulcer.

4. **Two days later, you are on rounds and notice that A. S.'s serum creatinine has increased from 1.2 mg/dL to 2.4 mg/dL. Which of the following statements regarding his antimicrobial therapy is true? (He is currently receiving meropenem 2 g IVPB every 8 hours and gentamicin 160 mg IVPB every 12 hours.)**

    a. **Change regimen to piperacillin/tazobactam plus tobramycin**
    b. **Consider discontinuation of gentamicin**
    c. **Recommend that the meropenem dose/interval be adjusted to 1 g every 12 hours**
    d. **Change regimen to ciprofloxacin**
    e. **Both b and c**

Answer e is correct. A. S.'s CrCl has decreased from 56 mL/min to 28 mL/min (using the Cockcroft-Gault equation and ideal body weight). As aminoglycosides can cause nephrotoxicity, it is reasonable to recommend that the gentamicin be discontinued (b). Meropenem is renally eliminated, and the manufacturer recommends a dosage adjustment at CrCl of 26 to 50 mL/min to 1 g every 12 hours (c). Failure to adjust dosage may increase the risk of adverse effects, including seizures. Imipenem/cilastatin has a higher risk of seizures than meropenem; however, a risk exists with meropenem. On the basis of susceptibilities, *Pseudomonas* is sensitive to piperacillin, but tobramycin is an aminoglycoside, which can still worsen A. S.'s renal function. It would not be a reasonable option to change therapy to piperacillin plus tobramycin (a). It is also not reasonable to change the regimen to ciprofloxacin alone as the patient requires anaerobic coverage for his perforated ulcer (d).

5. **A physician orders ceftazidime 2 g IVPB every 8 hours for a patient with an *Enterobacter* species nosocomial pneumonia. Susceptibility testing shows that the pathogen is susceptible to ceftazidime. The patient initially responds to therapy but subsequently worsens. What has potentially happened?**

   a. ***Enterobacter*** **possesses an inducible beta-lactamase gene (type I beta-lactamase enzyme) that in the presence of a beta-lactam induces this enzyme.**
   b. **Alteration in DNA gyrase is causing resistance.**
   c. **Underdosage of the ceftazidime has induced resistance.**
   d. **Nonadherence**
   e. **Ceftazidime does not penetrate into the lung.**

   Answer a is correct. *Enterobacter* species may contain inducible beta-lactamase genes that in the presence of ceftazidime (a third-generation cephalosporin) may be induced (a). Both *Klebsiella* and *Enterobacter* species may contain extended-spectrum beta-lactamases. In these cases, the carbapenems appear to be first-line therapy. Therefore, what shows to be susceptible in the lab is not actually susceptible in vivo. Beta-lactam agents are cell wall active agents; therefore, alterations in the DNA gyrase of organisms will not affect their activity against an organism (b). Quinolones act on DNA gyrase. Although underdosing may promote the emergence of resistant organisms, ceftazidime at a dose of 2 g every 8 hours is not underdosed (c). Patient nonadherence rarely plays a role in the inpatient setting (d). Ceftazidime has adequate lung penetration (e).

6. **Which of the following oral antibiotics could be used to complete treatment of pneumonia for A. S. as an outpatient?**

   a. **Meropenem**
   b. **Cefuroxime**
   c. **Amoxicillin/clavulanate**
   d. **Ciprofloxacin**
   e. **Moxifloxacin**

   Answer d is correct. On the basis of culture and susceptibility data, ciprofloxacin (d) is the only listed agent that is active against the *P. aeruginosa*. Meropenem does not come as an oral agent (a). Cefuroxime (b), amoxicillin/clavulanate (c), and moxifloxacin (e) do not have activity against *P. aeruginosa*.

BIBLIOGRAPHY

American Thoracic Society; Infectious Diseases Society of America. Guidelines for the management of adults with hospital-acquired, ventilator-associated, and healthcare-associated pneumonia. *Am J Respir Crit Care Med.* 2005;171(4):388-416.

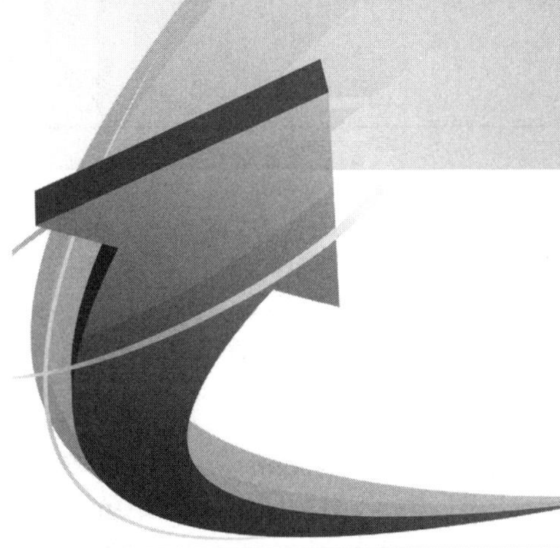

CASE 2.12
Influenza | Level 2

SELF-ASSESSMENT ANSWERS

1. What agents are recommended by the Centers for Disease Control and Prevention (CDC) for treatment and/or prophylaxis against influenza?

Oral oseltamivir and inhaled zanamivir are recommended for both prevention and treatment of influenza A and B. In 2014, the U.S. Food and Drug Administration approved Rapivab® (peramivir) to treat influenza infection in adults, but it is available only in IV form. Amantadine and rimantadine are adamantanes, and they are not currently recommended by the CDC for the prevention or treatment of influenza A because of widespread adamantane resistance among currently circulating influenza A viruses. The adamantanes are not active against influenza B.

2. What is the mechanism of action of the neuraminidase inhibitors?

Neuraminidase catalyzes the hydrolysis of terminal sialic acid residues from newly formed virions and host cell receptors, allowing virions to be released from the infected cell. Hence, a neuraminidase inhibitor blocks the release of new influenza A and B virions.

3. Develop an appropriate treatment plan for T. D. at this time.

Of the available treatment options, oseltamivir 75 mg po bid for 5 days would be the most appropriate initial choice for the treatment of influenza A in this patient. Longer durations may be considered for patients who remain severely ill after 5 days of therapy. Zanamivir 10 mg inhaled bid for 5 days is another appropriate option. Peramivir is also an option, but it is available only via the IV route. Prophylaxis dosing may be administered for 7 (CDC, 2012 or American Academy of Pediatrics, 2013) to 10 days (manufacturer recommendation).

4. What, if any, clinical benefit is likely to be seen by starting antiviral treatment in T. D. at this time?

Treatment of influenza with an anti-influenza agent will shorten the duration of the illness by an average of 1 day when started within 48 hours of symptoms. Clinical benefit is greatest, the earlier the antiviral medication is initiated. Early antiviral treatment will also reduce the risk of complications from influenza such as pneumonia and death. However, treatment will not prevent influenza from occurring in subsequent seasons and will not eliminate the need for future vaccinations in subsequent flu seasons. Antiviral treatment might benefit patients with severe, complicated, or progressive illness, and in hospitalized patients when started after 48 hours of the onset of symptoms.

5. Which of the following patients would be an appropriate candidate for vaccination with a standard dose, inactivated influenza vaccine?

a. A 3-month-old healthy infant

b. A 45-year-old man with a history of an anaphylactic reaction to the inactivated influenza vaccine

c. A 28-year-old pregnant woman

d. A 15-year-old with a moderate-to-severe illness associated with fever

e. A 68-year-old woman who developed Guillain-Barré syndrome within 6 weeks of receiving the influenza vaccine in the past

Answer c is correct. The standard dose, inactivated influenza vaccine is approved for use in pregnant women, while the quadrivalent, live attenuated influenza vaccine is contraindicated in pregnant women. The inactivated influenza vaccine is not approved for use in children less than 6 months of age (a). A previous severe allergic reaction to influenza vaccine is a contraindication to future receipt of the vaccine (b). Patients who have developed Guillain-Barré syndrome within 6 weeks of receiving influenza vaccine in the past generally should not receive the vaccination again (e). The influenza vaccine is not recommended for patients with a moderate-to-severe febrile illness (d) because the vaccine may not be as effective during the acute illness.

6. Which patient groups are candidates for the quadrivalent, live attenuated influenza vaccine?

The live attenuated influenza vaccine is indicated for healthy, nonpregnant persons aged 2 to 49 years. Contraindications to the quadrivalent, live attenuated influenza vaccine include pregnancy, immunosuppression, history of an egg allergy, and patients who have taken influenza antiviral medications within the previous 48 hours. Precautions for the live attenuated influenza vaccine are moderate or acute illness, a patient history of Guillain-Barré syndrome within 6 weeks of vaccination, and patients with chronic medical conditions such as chronic lung diseases, diabetes, renal or hepatic diseases, hematologic diseases, neurologic diseases, and metabolic diseases.

BIBLIOGRAPHY

Centers for Disease Control and Prevention. Influenza Antiviral Medications: Summary for Clinicians. http://www.cdc.gov/flu/professionals/antivirals/summary-clinicians.htm. Accessed February 21, 2015.

Centers for Disease Control and Prevention. Influenza. http://www.cdc.gov/flu/index.htm. Accessed February 21, 2015.

Centers for Disease Control and Prevention. Immunization Schedules. http://www.cdc.gov/vaccines/schedules/index.html. Accessed February 21, 2015.

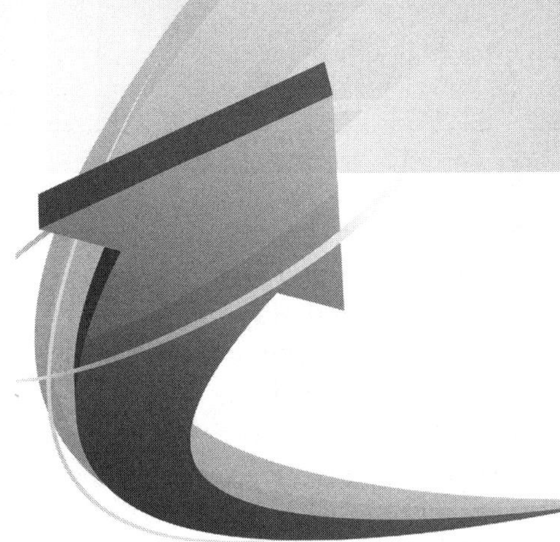

CASE 2.13
Tuberculosis | Level 3

SELF-ASSESSMENT ANSWERS

1. On the basis of the information provided, tuberculin screening skin tests (PPD) should be given to which family members?

The PPD skin test (Mantoux test) is used to detect *Mycobacterium tuberculosis* (MTB) infections in individuals with subclinical disease (latent infection). Infection can lead to positive PPD reactions within 6 to 8 weeks of exposure. Those individuals with a history of significant exposure to a known case of active TB should be screened for infection using the PPD skin test. In this case, because M. B.'s husband, grown daughter, grandchildren, sister, and her sister's family all have significant exposure, they all should be screened with the PPD skin test.

2. The patient's husband has a positive reaction within 48 hours of administration of a PPD skin test. What is considered a positive reaction of a PPD skin test?

A reaction of greater than 5 mm to 5 TU Mantoux test after 48 hours is considered positive for those patients with recent close contact with infectious TB cases and also for patients who are HIV positive, persons with fibrotic changes consistent with old healed TB, patients with organ transplants, and other immunosuppressed patients. A reaction of greater than 10 mm is positive for patients who are recent arrivals from high-prevalence countries, IV drug users, residents or employees of high-risk congregate settings, mycobacteriology lab personnel, persons with clinical conditions that place them at risk, children less than 4 years old, and adolescents exposed to adults in the high-risk category. A reaction of greater than 15 mm is positive for patients with no TB risk factors. The area of induration measures a patient with a positive TB reaction. Erythema is not considered. Tests must be read in 48 to 72 hours for an accurate reading.

3. Which one of the following statements is *false* regarding the QuantiFERON-TB Gold In-Tube test (QFT-GIT)?

a. It may be used to diagnose both latent and active TB infections.

b. QFT-GIT should be used in place of a PPD skin test, but *not* in addition to a PPD skin test.

- **c. A prior BCG (Bacillus Calmette–Guérin) vaccination does *not* cause a false-positive result.**
- **d. The patient must return to clinic within 48 to 72 hours to assess the reaction.**
- **e. QFT-GIT is not preferred over a PPD in children less than 5 years of age.**

Answer d is correct. In 2007, the QFT-GIT test was approved by the FDA for use as a diagnostic test for both latent and active *M. tuberculosis* infections (a). Current CDC guidelines state that the QFT-GIT test may be used in place of a PPD "in all situations in which CDC recommends TST (tuberculin skin testing) as an aid in diagnosing *M. tuberculosis* infection" (b). Unlike the PPD skin test, the QFT-GIT results may be available within 24 hours and don't require a return visit to the clinic (d). False positives do not occur if the patient has had a previous BCG vaccine (c). The CDC has specific recommendations available as to certain situations in which either the PPD or the QFT-GIT tests would be preferred over the other (e). One example included is that in children under the age of 5, the PPD test is preferred over QFT-GIT due to its lack of data in this population.

4. What is an initial appropriate treatment recommendation for M. B.'s pulmonary TB disease? In addition to the specific anti-TB regimen selected, what other therapy should be considered for M. B. at this time?

For initial empiric treatment of TB, a four-drug regimen consisting of isoniazid, rifampin, pyrazinamide, and ethambutol (or streptomycin) is recommended. The short course or 6-month regimen is preferred for therapy of TB. This consists of 2 months of isoniazid, rifampin, pyrazinamide, and ethambutol (or streptomycin) followed by 4 months of isoniazid and rifampin. TB should be treated with at least two agents that the organism is susceptible to in order to prevent the emergence of resistance. The 6-month course is the shortest duration of effective therapy. Treatment should be continued for at least 6 months from the time of a negative smear and culture. If pyrazinamide is not included in the initial regimen, treatment should continue for 9 months. Directly observed therapy (DOT) is recommended for treatment. Many clinicians consider adding daily doses of pyridoxine (25 to 50 mg) in patients who are treated with isoniazid to offset potential neurological side effects of isoniazid therapy.

5. M. B.'s liver function tests increase to two times the original concentrations after 1 month of therapy with isoniazid, rifampin, pyrazinamide, and ethambutol. M. B. does not have any complaints regarding her drug therapy, other than having to take so many drugs in a single day. Which of the following should *not* be a recommended change to her drug therapy?

- **a. Decrease the dose of isoniazid to half the starting dose; discontinue the rifampin.**
- **b. Interview the patient monthly for symptoms of hepatotoxicity.**
- **c. Inform the patient of symptoms of hepatotoxicity and tell her to report these to her doctor if they occur.**
- **d. Maintain the original doses of isoniazid, rifampin, and pyrazinamide.**
- **e. Monitor liver function tests for the entire course of therapy.**

Answer a is correct. In the presence of symptoms, elevation of liver function tests to three times the normal range may warrant discontinuation of drug at least temporarily. If no symptoms are present, continuation of medications until the liver function tests are over five times the normal range may be reasonable (a). Choices b through e can be recommended.

6. One of M. B.'s grandchildren has a positive reaction to the PPD skin test. What therapy, if any, should be initiated in this 6-year-old male who is otherwise healthy and without clinical evidence of TB?

Prophylaxis (treatment of latent TB infection) with isoniazid is recommended for those individuals who have a new conversion of a PPD and no other clinical manifestations of TB. The appropriate dose of isoniazid is 10 to 15 mg/kg/day (maximum dose 300 mg) for 9 months). Moxifloxacin should not be used in pediatric patients. Rifampin can be used as an alternative to isoniazid. Ethambutol has not been used as a single agent for TB prophylaxis.

BIBLIOGRAPHY

Centers for Disease Control and Prevention. TB Guidelines. http://www.cdc.gov/tb/publications/guidelines/list_date.htm. Accessed February 21, 2015.

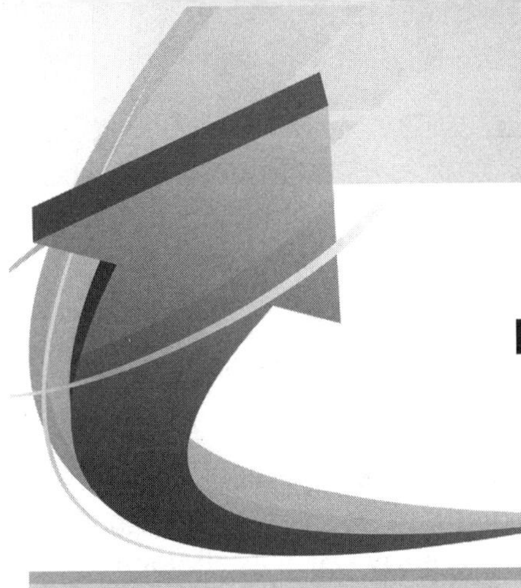

CASE 2.14
Healthcare-Associated Pneumonia | Level 3

SELF-ASSESSMENT ANSWERS

1. The medical resident needs to initiate therapy for V. T. and asks if he should administer ceftriaxone alone or a combination of levofloxacin and vancomycin. What is the best response to the resident?

V. T. is diagnosed with healthcare-associated pneumonia (HCAP). Ceftriaxone is a commonly used single-agent therapy for patients with hospital-acquired pneumonia and no known risk factors, but it is not appropriate for HCAP therapy. Levofloxacin and vancomycin are appropriate if an antipseudomonal cephalosporin, antipseudomonal carbapenem, or beta-lactam/beta-lactam inhibitor is added to therapy. A three-drug combination antibiotic regimen is warranted as empiric therapy for HCAP in patients with risk factors for multidrug resistant pathogens. V. T. has risk factors of antimicrobial use in the past 3 months and potential group home residential situation.

2. Which antibiotics potentially used for HCAP have postantibiotic effects?

Aminoglycosides and fluoroquinolones exhibit postantibiotic effect against gram-negative bacilli. Beta-lactams usually have little to no postantibiotic effects. Carbapenems are an exception to this as they have postantibiotic effects against gram-negative bacilli.

3. What if you had a patient with pneumonia and *Acinetobacter* spp. was the causative pathogen, what antibiotics are the most active against this species?

Acinetobacter spp. has native resistance to several antibiotic classes. If *Acinetobacter* spp. was a causative pathogen in pneumonia, carbapenems, ampicillin/sulbactam, polymyxin, and colistin are the most active antimicrobials. A carbapenem is an appropriate empiric therapy. The activity of ampicillin/sulbactam against *Acinetobacter* comes from the sulbactam component. Nephrotoxic effects of polymyxin may limit its use depending on patient factors; however, aerosolized therapy may be considered.

4. What should the clinician do if the patient is not responding to initial therapy?

If a patient is not responding to initial therapy, the organism, diagnosis, and complications should be considered. First, question if the patient has a different organism than originally expected or if the patient has an inadequate antimicrobial therapy. Ensure the drug can reach the infection site in the body, considering issues such as absorption or chelation. Could other diagnoses be relevant, or could complications have occurred? Host, pathogen, and therapeutic factors should all be questioned and considered.

5. In evaluating his vaccine record, does V. T. need any immunizations at this time or in the future?

V. T. should receive the Tdap vaccine at this time. If available, he should also receive the inactivated influenza vaccine annually. V. T. should not receive the live attenuated influenza vaccine due to his pulmonary disease. However, because of his pulmonary disease, he should receive the PPSV23 vaccine at this time. One year from now he should receive the PCV13, and 5 years from now he should receive another PPSV23. Once he turns 60 years of age, he should receive the zoster vaccine.

6. If V. T. had a history of experiencing shortness of breath with amoxicillin use, what medication would have been an appropriate treatment for the presumed acute pharyngitis?

If V. T. had a history of a severe allergic reaction with amoxicillin, then it would have been best to use an alternative such as clindamycin, azithromycin, or clarithromycin to treat the acute pharyngitis. Penicillins and cephalosporins should be avoided. First-generation cephalosporins could be used if the patient had experienced a non-IgE-mediated reaction.

BIBLIOGRAPHY

American Thoracic Society; Infectious Diseases Society of America. Guidelines for the management of adults with hospital-acquired, ventilator-associated, and healthcare-associated pneumonia. *Am J Respir Crit Care Med.* 2005;171(4):388-416.

Centers for Disease Control and Prevention. Immunization schedules. http://www.cdc.gov/vaccines/schedules/index.html. Accessed February 19, 2015.

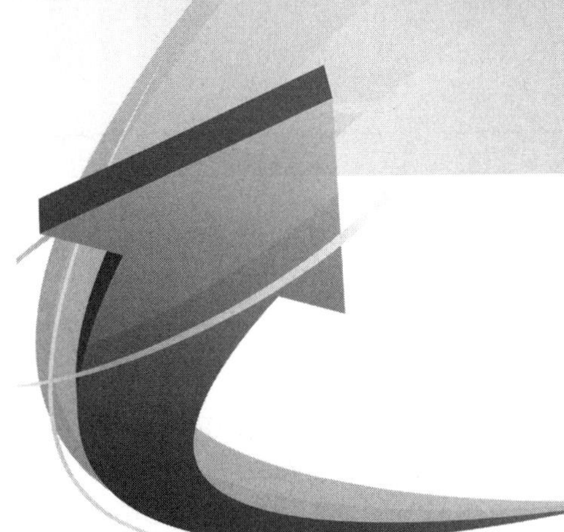

CASE 2.15
Neonatal Sepsis | Level 1

SELF-ASSESSMENT ANSWERS

1. What organisms are common causes of early-onset sepsis in a neonate? What organisms are common causes of late-onset sepsis in a neonate? What are the transmission methods of the organisms for early-onset and late-onset sepsis?

Early-onset sepsis is defined as blood or cerebrospinal fluid culture-proven infection occurring in a newborn younger than 7 days of age (usually acquired intrapartum). Some clinicians define early-onset occurring during the first 3 days of life. Group B *Streptococcus*, the primary pathogen causing early-onset sepsis, is a gram-positive cocci organism in pairs or chains. *Escherichia coli* is a gram-negative rod organism that is a common cause of early-onset sepsis. In addition to group B *Streptococcus* and *E. coli,* other causes of early-onset sepsis include *Haemophilus influenzae, Klebsiella* spp., *Enterobacter* spp., and *Listeria monocytogenes,* which is a gram-positive bacilli organism.

Staphylococcus epidermidis, or coagulase-negative *Staphylococcus,* is a gram-positive organism that is a common cause of late-onset sepsis in the newborn. *Staphylococcus aureus, E. coli, Enterococcus, Klebsiella* spp., *Enterobacter* spp., and *Candida* spp. can be a cause of late-onset sepsis as well. Late-onset sepsis is usually acquired postnatally from the environment. Coagulase-negative *Staphylococcus* is primarily from catheter-related infections.

2. What are risk factors for early-onset sepsis and late-onset sepsis in a neonate?

Risk factors for early-onset sepsis in a neonate include preterm birth, maternal colonization with group B *Streptococcus*, rupture of membranes greater than 18 hours, and maternal signs or symptoms of intra-amniotic infection. Other risk factors include ethnicity (African-American female mothers), low socioeconomic status, male gender, and low APGAR scores.

Risk factors for late-onset sepsis include prematurity, especially in infants with prolonged hospitalization. Other risk factors include low birth weight, previous antimicrobial exposure, poor hand hygiene, and the use of central venous catheters.

3. **Describe the mechanism of actions of gentamicin and ampicillin. Why are these antibiotics recommended for empiric use in early-onset sepsis?**

Gentamicin is an aminoglycoside antibiotic and binds to the 30S and 50S ribosomal subunit. This causes an inhibition of protein synthesis and results in a faulty cell wall membrane. Ampicillin is a penicillin antibiotic and causes cell death by binding to penicillin-binding proteins and affecting the cell wall. Ampicillin and gentamicin is the common regimen selected for early-onset sepsis as both antibiotics cover the most common pathogens. Ampicillin is the drug of choice for *Listeria*, and both drugs are synergistic for group B *Streptococcus*. The majority of *E. coli* isolates in the United States are resistant to ampicillin, but sensitivity patterns to aminoglycosides are highly susceptible. Some institutions may replace the gentamicin with cefotaxime; however, concerns exist with the potential development of resistant pathogens due to third-generation cephalosporin use within an ICU. In addition, the risk of invasive candidiasis increases with prolonged use of third-generation cephalosporins.

4. **Gentamicin serum levels return for Baby Girl Smith. The trough is 0.9 mcg/mL, and the peak is 7.8 mcg/mL. Levels were all drawn appropriately. How would you adjust her current dose?**

Gentamicin has a goal trough less than 2 mcg/mL and a goal peak 4 to 8 mcg/mL. No change is needed for the current dose.

5. **At what time frame can discontinuing antibiotics in Baby Girl Smith be considered if she shows no signs of illness, feeds well, and cultures are negative?**

Antibiotics may be discontinued if the patient shows no signs of illness, is feeding well, and if the cultures are negative for 48 hours. Ninety-five percent of neonates with a group B streptococcal infection will show signs and symptoms of illness within the first 24 hours.

6. **Baby Girl Smith's blood and CSF cultures return positive for group B *Streptococcus*. What alterations do you recommend for antibiotic treatment and duration of therapy, if any?**

Infants with group B *Streptococcus* in the blood and CSF should be treated with ampicillin and gentamicin initially. Antibiotic de-escalation can occur once susceptibilities are known. Ampicillin should be dosed at 100 mg/kg/dose every 12 hours for bacteremia and every 8 hours for meningitis in a preterm infant of her age and weight. Because Baby Girl Smith's CSF was positive, her ampicillin dose should remain the same, but the regimen should be adjusted to every 8 hours. Baby Girl Smith's gentamicin levels were within range so no adjustments were necessary. Uncomplicated meningitis with group B *Streptococcus* should be treated for a minimum of 14 days. Confirmed group B streptococcal sepsis only needs to be treated for 10 days duration.

BIBLIOGRAPHY

Polin RA; Committee on Fetus and Newborn. Management of neonates with suspected or proven early-onset bacterial sepsis. *Pediatrics.* 2012;129(5):1006-15.

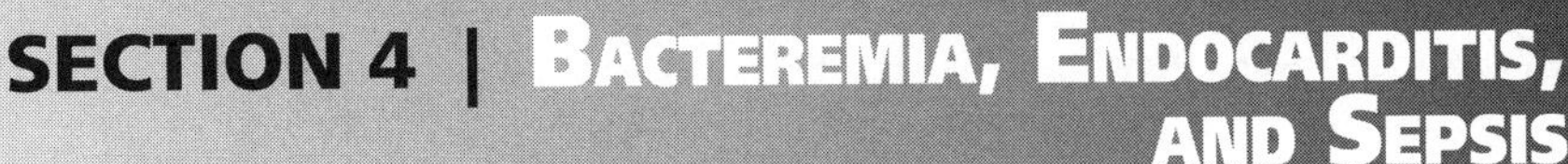
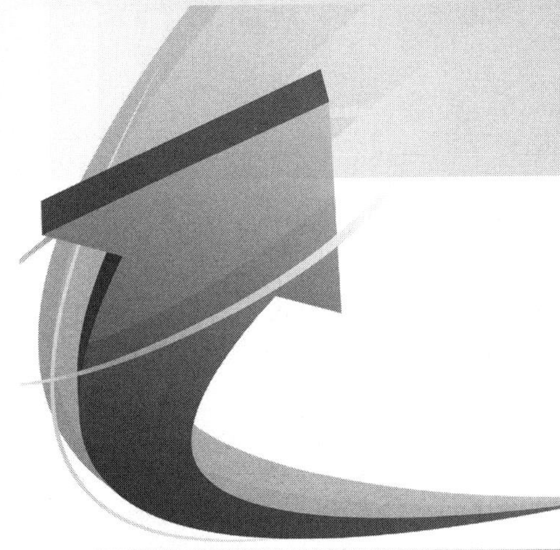

CASE 2.16
Infective Endocarditis—Viridans Group Streptococci | Level 1

SELF-ASSESSMENT ANSWERS

1. **Which of the symptoms exhibited by R. R. would be included as a Duke criteria contributing to the diagnosis of infective endocarditis?**

   Multiple blood cultures with an organism associated with endocarditis such as viridans group streptococci and a positive echocardiogram showing vegetation are major Duke criteria. A predisposing heart condition such as mitral valve prolapse and fever greater than 38°C are minor Duke criteria.

2. **Prior to receiving microbiology blood culture results, which pathogens would you consider when selecting empiric treatment options for this patient with suspected infective endocarditis?**

   Staphylococci occur in approximately 42% of the cases and are now the most common form of infective endocarditis. *S. aureus* is the predominant pathogen in staphylococcal cases involving native valves. Streptococci occur in 40% of cases; however, infective endocarditis caused by *S. pneumoniae* is very rare. Enterococci occur in 11% of cases of infective endocarditis. The balance is distributed over many more rare etiologies; however, *Candida* species, *E. coli,* and *P. aeruginosa* make up fewer than 5% of cases combined, so they are all very rare causes.

3. **What would be the best choice for empiric treatment of the two most likely pathogens for infective endocarditis in this patient? What treatment duration is warranted?**

   Both penicillin G and ceftriaxone are recommended for infective endocarditis caused by streptococci but are not recommended for staphylococci due to suboptimal activity. Treatment duration should be 4 weeks of IV therapy. Gentamicin may be added for synergy, and, if so, the treatment duration may be shortened to 2 weeks. Vancomycin would be an appropriate empiric choice until full identification and susceptibilities are available because it is active against streptococci, staphylococci, and susceptible strains of enterococci or for patients who cannot tolerate penicillin or ceftriaxone.

4. **What if the MIC of the viridans group streptococci was greater than 0.5 mcg/mL, resulting in a penicillin-resistant strain?**

   If a penicillin-resistant strain (MIC of greater than 0.5 mcg/mL) had grown from the culture, treatment should include IV penicillin or ceftriaxone administered for 4 weeks with the addition of IV gentamicin during the first 2 weeks of treatment.

5. **What would be the best antibiotic prophylaxis recommendation for a patient with a history of infective endocarditis undergoing an invasive dental procedure?**

   One dose of oral amoxicillin is the best recommendation for infective endocarditis prophylaxis. Clindamycin is recommended only for patients unable to tolerate penicillin. IV therapies such as ceftriaxone or vancomycin are recommended only in situations where patients are unable to take oral medication.

6. **If the physician believes this patient experienced a penicillin-induced, nonanaphylactoid-type allergic reaction during the patient's last admission, which antibiotic would you recommend for treatment at this admission?**

   Cephalosporins such as cefazolin may be safe for patients with a history of nonanaphylactoid reactions to penicillin, but they should be avoided in patients with anaphylactoid-type hypersensitivity to beta-lactams. Vancomycin should be used in cases where the use of beta-lactams has been ruled out. Risk of anaphylaxis exists on rechallenge to penicillins, and skin testing should be completed for a patient with a positive culture for oxacillin-susceptible staphylococci and questionable history of immediate-type hypersensitivity to penicillin.

BIBLIOGRAPHY

Baddour LM, Wilson WR, Bayer AS, et al. Infective endocarditis diagnosis, antimicrobial therapy, and management of complications: a statement for healthcare professionals from the Committee on Rheumatic Fever, Endocarditis, and Kawasaki Disease, Council on Cardiovascular Disease in the Young, and the Councils on Clinical Cardiology, Stroke, and Cardiovascular Surgery and Anesthesia, American Heart Association *Circulation.* 2005;111(23):e394-434.

Wilson W, Taubert KA, Gewitz M, et al. Prevention of infective endocarditis: guidelines from the American Heart Association Rheumatic Fever, Endocarditis, and Kawasaki Disease Committee, Council on Cardiovascular Disease in the Young, and the Council on Clinical Cardiology, Council on Cardiovascular Surgery and Anesthesia, and the Quality of Care and Outcomes Research Interdisciplinary Working Group. *Circulation.* 2007;116(15):1736-54.

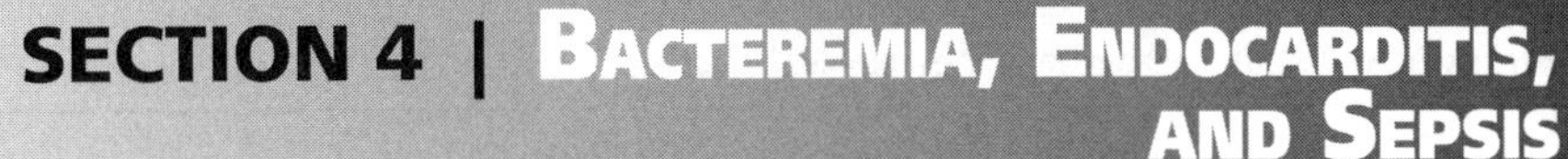

CASE 2.17
Catheter-Related Bloodstream Infection—Antibiotic Resistance | Level 2

SELF-ASSESSMENT ANSWERS

1. **Suppose the organism isolated in M. R.'s blood cultures returned as susceptible to oxacillin but resistant to penicillin G. Which of the following would be the most likely mechanism of resistance?**

   a. **Production of penicillinase**
   b. **Production of a penicillin efflux pump**
   c. **Alteration of penicillin-binding protein 2a**
   d. **Alteration of DNA gyrase**
   e. **Loss of a porin channel in the outer membrane**

   Answer a is correct. Oxacillin is a penicillinase-resistant penicillin. Choice b is incorrect because *S. aureus* does not produce penicillin efflux pumps. Choice c is incorrect because this is the mechanism of resistance for MRSA. Choice d is incorrect because this is a fluoroquinolone mechanism of resistance. Choice e is incorrect because gram-positive organisms do not have an outer membrane.

2. **Suppose the organism isolated in M. R.'s blood cultures returned as susceptible to vancomycin but resistant to oxacillin. Which of the following would be the most likely mechanism of resistance?**

   a. **Change from D-ala-D-ala to D-ala-D-lactate**
   b. **Alteration of penicillin-binding protein 2a**
   c. **Production of an extended-spectrum beta-lactamase**
   d. **Efflux of beta-lactam antibiotics**
   e. **Alteration of the 50S ribosomal subunit**

   Answer b is correct. Alteration of penicillin-binding protein 2a (PBP2a) is correct because an oxacillin-resistant, vancomycin-susceptible *S. aureus* isolate can be labeled as MRSA. The mechanism of methicillin resistance is an alteration in PBP2, which prevents all beta-lactam antibiotics from binding to the site of action. Choice a is incorrect because this is the vancomycin resistance mechanism. Vancomycin binds to D-ala-D-ala. Choice c is incorrect because staphylococci do not produce ESBLs. Choice d is incorrect because penicillin efflux pumps are not a resistance mechanism. Choice e is incorrect because an alteration of the 50S subunit only affects the activity of protein synthesis inhibitors.

3. **Suppose the organism isolated in M. R.'s blood cultures returned as MSSA susceptible to clindamycin and quinupristin/dalfopristin but resistant to erythromycin. Which of the following would be the most likely mechanism of resistance?**

   a. **Change from D-ala-D-ala to D-ala-D-lactate**
   b. **Alteration of penicillin-binding protein 2a**
   c. **Production of an extended-spectrum beta-lactamase**
   d. **Efflux of macrolide antibiotics**
   e. **Alteration of the 50S ribosomal subunit**

   Answer d is correct. Efflux of macrolide antibiotics is correct because a macrolide efflux pump would only cause resistance to erythromycin. Choice a is incorrect because it is the vancomycin resistance mechanism. Choice b is incorrect because a PBP2a mutation is the MRSA mechanism of resistance. Choice c is incorrect because staphylococci do not produce ESBLs. Choice e is incorrect because an alteration in the 50S subunit would cause resistance to macrolides (erythromycin), lincosamide (clindamycin), and streptogramins (quinupristin/dalfopristin).

4. **Suppose the organism isolated in M. R.'s blood cultures returned with a susceptibility profile suggesting a community-associated MRSA strain. Which antibiotic would be most appropriate for M. R. and at what dosing regimen? Does the catheter need to be removed?**

   According to the 2009 IDSA *Clinical Practice Guidelines for the Management of Intravascular Catheter-Related Infections*, IV vancomycin is the preferred agent despite the fact that CA-MRSA may be susceptible to drugs such as ciprofloxacin, clindamycin, and erythromycin. According to the 2009 ASHP/IDSA/SIDP *Therapeutic Monitoring of Vancomycin in Adult Patients*, a loading dose of 25 to 30 mg/kg (based on actual body weight) can be used to facilitate rapid attainment of target troughs in seriously ill patients. In addition, doses of 15 to 20 mg/kg (based on actual body weight) given every 8 to 12 hours are recommended for most patients with normal renal function.

   Loading dose = 25 mg/kg × 102 kg = 2,550 mg provided over at least 2 hours, consider pretreating with an antihistamine.

   Maintenance dose = 15 mg/kg × 102 kg = 1,530 mg either every 8 or 12 hours. The catheter should be removed.

5. **The third-year medical student asks you if antibiotic lock therapy could be used to treat this patient. How do you respond?**

   According to the 2009 IDSA *Clinical Practice Guidelines for the Management of Intravascular Catheter-Related Infections*, antibiotic lock therapy is indicated for patients with catheter-related blood stream infections that involve long-term catheters and when no signs of exit site or tunnel infection are identified. It is also indicated for patients when catheter salvage is the goal. Antibiotic lock therapy should be used with systemic therapy, not alone. Dwell times should be maximized between drug administration times and flushes.

6. **Which of the following strategies would be most effective for preventing future catheter-related bloodstream infections in M. R.?**

   a. **Changing the catheter site to the internal jugular vein**
   b. **Administering IV vancomycin for prophylaxis**
   c. **Flushing the catheter daily with heparin**
   d. **Using an inline filter when infusing drugs**
   e. **Using aseptic technique when inserting a new catheter**

   Answer e is correct. According to the 2011 *Guidelines for the Prevention of Intravascular Catheter-Related Infections,* aseptic technique is the primary general strategy for preventing catheter-related infections. Choice a is incorrect because catheters inserted in the internal jugular vein have been associated with a higher risk of infection compared to subclavian sites. Choice b is incorrect because systemic vancomycin is an independent risk factor for acquiring vancomycin-resistant enterococci and has not been shown to reduce catheter-related infections in adults. Choices c and d are incorrect because these strategies do not reduce infection. These are recommended because heparin reduces the rate of thrombosis and inline filters may reduce the rate of infusion-related phlebitis.

BIBLIOGRAPHY

Mermel LA, Allon M, Bouza E, et al. Clinical practice guidelines for the management of intravascular catheter-related infections: 2009 update by the Infectious Diseases Society of America. *Clin Infect Dis.* 2009;49(1):1-45.

O'Grady NP, Alexander M, Burns LA, et al. Guidelines for the prevention of intravascular catheter-related infections. *Clin Infect Dis.* 2011; 52(9):e162-93.

Rybak M, Lomaestro B, Rotschafer JC, et al. Therapeutic monitoring of vancomycin in adult patients: a consensus review of the American Society of Health-System Pharmacists, the Infectious Diseases Society of America, and the Society of Infectious Diseases Pharmacists. *Am J Health-Syst Pharm.* 2009;86(1):82-98.

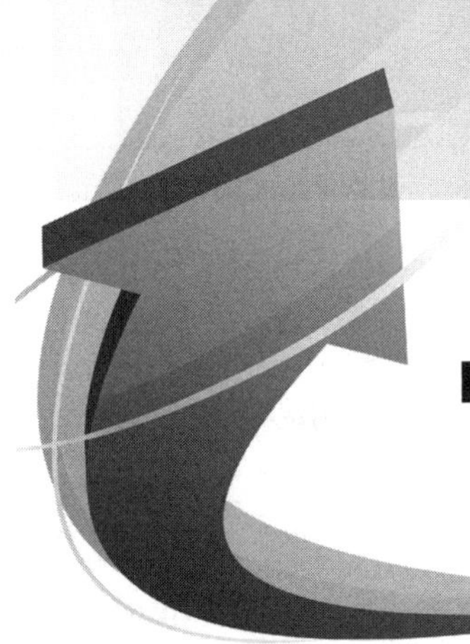

CASE 2.18
Infective Endocarditis—*Staphylococcus* | Level 2

SELF-ASSESSMENT ANSWERS

1. What are risk factors for infective endocarditis from *Streptococcus, Staphylococcus,* and *Enterococcus* organisms?

Underlying cardiac abnormalities are the leading cause of streptococcal endocarditis. Endocarditis associated with poor dentition would also most frequently be caused by *Streptococcus. Staphylococcus aureus* endocarditis is the most common cause among IV drug abusers. Genitourinary manipulations in older men and obstetric procedures in younger women are most frequently associated with enterococcal endocarditis. Hospital-acquired infections are also a risk factor for *Staphylococcus* or *Enterococcus* infections.

2. Compare and contrast transesophageal echocardiogram (TEE) to transthoracic echocardiogram (TTE) for the evaluation of infective endocarditis.

TEE is a more invasive exam than TTE, and TEE is both a more sensitive and more costly exam to perform. TEE is also more sensitive in detecting vegetation in patients with prosthetic valves. Specificity is similar between the two tests. TEE would not be recommended as a first exam for populations where suspicion of infective endocarditis is relatively low or for patients that may not be able to tolerate the exam due to the more invasive nature.

3. If blood cultures identify methicillin-sensitive *Staphylococcus* in a patient with known or suspected infective endocarditis, what antibiotic therapy should be initiated?

Nafcillin or oxacillin plus gentamicin is the drug regimen of choice in patients with oxacillin-susceptible staphylococcal cultures per the current treatment guidelines. Some clinicians will preferentially use cefazolin due to a better ADR profile and fewer doses per day. Gentamicin is recommended as an optional addition to nafcillin or oxacillin in relevant treatment guidelines. Most clinicians are not comfortable with nafcillin alone until blood cultures show no growth, unless there is a compelling reason not to use gentamicin (e.g., patient cannot tolerate, renal insufficiency). Gentamicin is not recommended as sole therapy. For penicillin-allergic (nonanaphylactoid type) patients, cefazolin may be used. Due to penicillinase production, most *Staphylo-*

coccus species are generally resistant to penicillin G. Vancomycin is considered inferior to a beta-lactam for treating oxacillin-susceptible *Staphylococcus*.

4. What is the recommended gentamicin dose for endocarditis caused by methicillin-sensitive *Staphylococcus aureus* (MSSA) in a patient with normal renal function? What are the target gentamicin peak and trough concentrations in the treatment of gram-positive cocci endocarditis?

Gentamicin initial dosing of 1 mg/kg every 8 hours infused over 30 to 60 minutes is the recommended dose for staphylococcal endocarditis. Doses are further adjusted based on follow-up serum peak and trough concentrations and changing renal function. Gentamicin is recommended as an adjunctive agent for synergy against gram-positive organisms. For synergistic dosing of gentamicin, the target peak serum concentrations are 3 to 4 mcg/mL. Trough target serum concentrations for gentamicin should always be less than or equal to 1 mcg/mL to minimize drug exposure.

5. The most recent microbiology sensitivity report noted growth of methicillin-resistant *Staphylococcus aureus* (MRSA), and the patient continues to have a low-grade fever. What drug regimen would you recommend to the prescribing physician?

MRSA is not susceptible to nafcillin, oxacillin, or cefazolin. Gentamicin is not appropriate as monotherapy for endocarditis. Vancomycin is the drug of choice for infective endocarditis caused by methicillin-resistant strains of *Staphylococcus*. Vancomycin is recommended to be dosed at 15 to 20 mg/kg/dose of actual body weight every 8 to 12 hours, not exceeding 2 g per dose, in patients with normal renal function. It should be infused over 60 to 90 minutes, and the dose should be adjusted to achieve trough concentrations 15 to 20 mcg/mL. In ill patients with serious infections such as endocarditis, a vancomycin loading dose of 25 to 30 mg/kg may be considered using a longer infusion time.

6. For which of the following patient factors would infective endocarditis prophylaxis be reasonable for a patient undergoing an invasive dental procedure where bleeding from gingival tissue is expected to occur?

a. Heart failure

b. Mitral valve prolapse without valve dysfunction

c. Atrial septal defect

d. Cardiac pacemaker

e. Previous endocarditis

Answer e is correct. The most recent guidelines for the prevention of infective endocarditis suggest that the potential complications with giving antibiotic prophylaxis outweigh the benefit when considering the low risk of acquisition of endocarditis through a transient bacteremia from an invasive dental procedure except in a few circumstances. A previous case of endocarditis (e) increases the risk of getting endocarditis again, and prophylaxis is recommended for that patient population. Cardiac conditions such as heart failure (a), mitral valve prolapse without valve dysfunction (b), atrial septal defects (c), and a cardiac pacemaker are not conditions for which prophylaxis is currently recommended.

BIBLIOGRAPHY

Baddour LM, Wilson WR, Bayer AS, et al. Infective endocarditis: diagnosis, antimicrobial therapy, and management of complications: a statement for healthcare professionals from the Committee on Rheumatic Fever, Endocarditis, and Kawasaki Disease, Council on Cardiovascular Disease in the Young, and the Councils on Clinical Cardiology, Stroke, and Cardiovascular Surgery and Anesthesia, American Heart Association *Circulation*. 2005;111(23):e394-434.

Liu C, Bayer A, Cosgrove SE, et al. Clinical practice guidelines by the Infectious Diseases Society of America for the treatment of methicillin-resistant *Staphylococcus aureus* infections in adults and children. *Clin Infect Dis*. 2011;52(3):e18-55.

Wilson W, Taubert KA, Gewitz M, et al. Prevention of infective endocarditis: guidelines from the American Heart Association: a guideline from the American Heart Association Rheumatic Fever, Endocarditis, and

Kawasaki Disease Committee, Council on Cardiovascular Disease in the Young, and the Council on Clinical Cardiology, Council on Cardiovascular Surgery and Anesthesia, and the Quality of Care and Outcomes Research Interdisciplinary Working Group. *Circulation.* 2007;116(15):1736-54.

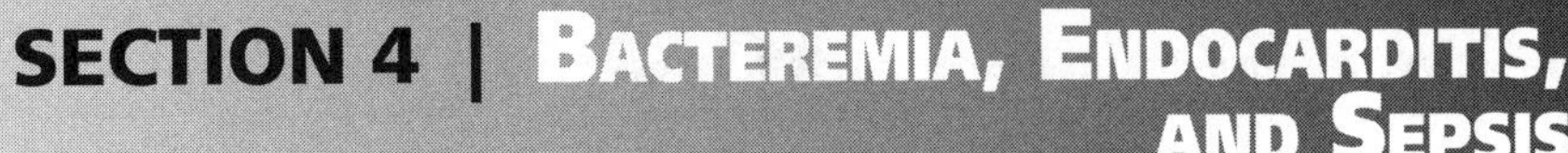

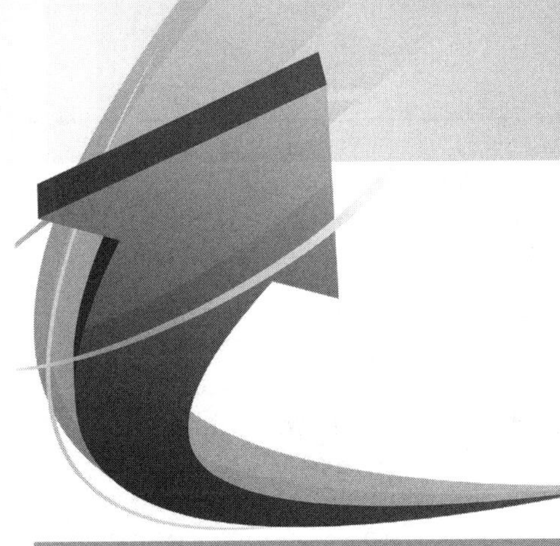

CASE 2.19
Bacteremia, Gram Positive | Level 2

SELF-ASSESSMENT ANSWERS

1. **An M4 medical student asks you about guidelines for preventing central catheter-related infections. Which of the following would be an appropriate recommendation?**

   a. **Promptly remove any intravascular catheter that is no longer essential.**

   b. **Change tunneled catheter site dressings every 2 days until the site has healed.**

   c. **Give a dose of prophylactic antibiotics 1 hour before catheter insertion.**

   d. **Replace the central venous catheter every 2 weeks.**

   e. **Use a vancomycin antibiotic lock solution for all idle central catheter ports.**

   Answer a is correct. The CDC's *Guidelines for the Prevention of Intravascular Catheter-Related Infections* outlines many strategies for preventing IV catheter-related infections. Under the section on Central Venous Catheters Recommendations, one of the recommendations is to remove intravascular catheter devices when no longer necessary (a). Choice b is incorrect as dressings should *not* be changed on tunneled or implanted catheters more than once a week until the insertion site has healed. Choice c is incorrect as pre-insertion prophylactic antibiotics are not recommended to be given routinely. Choice d is incorrect as central venous catheters are *not* routinely replaced. Choice e is incorrect as antibiotic lock solutions should be used only in special circumstances.

2. **What antimicrobial agents and duration should be used first line for bacteremia?**

   Vancomycin or daptomycin should be recommended for uncomplicated bacteremia for a duration of at least 2 weeks.

3. **The attending physician started M. C. on vancomycin therapy. When monitoring vancomycin serum concentrations, what is the recommended trough level range for the treatment of bacteremia?**

Vancomycin should be dosed at 15 to 20 mg/kg/dose (actual body weight) every 8 to 12 hours, not to exceed 2 g per dose, in patients with normal renal function. Daptomycin should be dosed at 6 mg/kg/dose IV once daily. Complicated bacteremia should be treated for 4 to 6 weeks. A higher daptomycin dose of 8 to 10 mg/kg/dose IV once daily is recommended by some experts and is being used in practice. A consensus statement from IDSA, ASHP, and SIDP recommends vancomycin dosing based on target serum trough levels no less than 10 mg/L for less serious infections and 15 to 20 mg/L for more serious infections such as bacteremia, osteomyelitis, meningitis, and hospital-acquired pneumonia.

4. You receive a call from M. C.'s nurse stating that M. C. became slightly hypotensive (110/60 mm Hg) and developed a rash on her trunk and arms when receiving her first dose of vancomycin. What actions do you recommend?

This type of reaction is not usually an allergic reaction but a reaction related to the rate of infusion. The best advice is to slow down the rate of the infusion.

5. By day 7 of therapy with vancomycin, M. C. is clinically stable, but a recent chemistry panel shows an increase in her serum creatinine to 1.9 mg/dL. Assuming that the bacteria was found to be methicillin-resistant *Staphylococcus aureus* (MRSA) and the patient was going to be continued on IV vancomycin, how would you empirically dose the drug in this patient?

The patient's renal function is approximately 25 mL/min based on the Cockcroft-Gault equation using her ideal body weight and serum creatinine of 1.9 mg/dL. Vancomycin 1,000 mg every 24 hours is correct because it is the appropriate interval, and the dose is approximately 15 mg/kg, which is the recommendation in the guidelines.

6. After 10 days on IV vancomycin, the medical fellow wants to convert this patient to oral vancomycin. He wants to know whether an oral formulation of vancomycin is available and what the most appropriate dose is for this patient. What is the best response?

Both oral capsule and solution forms of vancomycin are available. However, due to its poor absorption and very limited bioavailability outside the gastrointestinal tract, it cannot be used to treat systemic infections. Its only use is in the treatment of *C. difficile* pseudomembranous colitis.

7. If the bacteria causing the patient's infection are determined to be methicillin-sensitive *Staphylococcus aureus* (MSSA), what antibiotic would be the optimal choice for treatment?

Nafcillin, oxacillin, or cefazolin are the drugs of choice for this bacteria. Vancomycin will cover MSSA, but several studies have demonstrated that beta-lactam antibiotics are more effective than vancomycin for MSSA. Linezolid could be an option, but its bacteriostatic characteristics—rather than bactericidal—make it a less appealing choice. Ceftaroline covers MSSA but is not currently FDA approved for the treatment of bloodstream infections.

BIBLIOGRAPHY

Liu C, Bayer A, Cosgrove SE, et al. Clinical practice guidelines by the Infectious Diseases Society of America for the treatment of methicillin-resistant *Staphylococcus aureus* infections in adults and children. *Clin Infect Dis.* 2011;52(3):e18-55.

O'Grady NP, Alexander M, Burns LA, et al. Guidelines for the prevention of intravascular catheter-related infections. *Clin Infect Dis.* 2011;52(9):e162-93.

Rybak M, Lomaestro B, Rotschafer JC, et al. Therapeutic monitoring of vancomycin in adult patients: a consensus review of the American Society of Health-System Pharmacists, the Infectious Diseases Society of America, and the Society of Infectious Diseases Pharmacists. *Am J Health-Syst Pharm.* 2009;66(1):82-98.

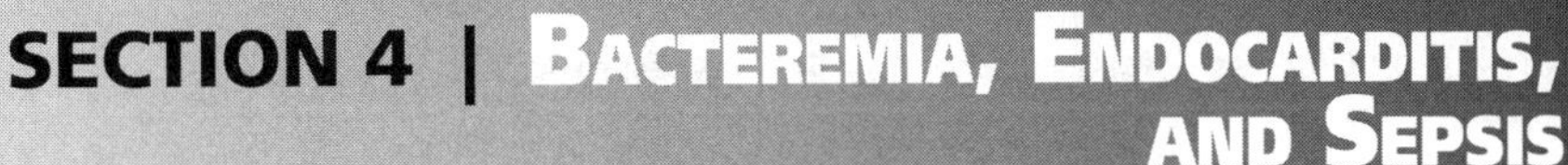

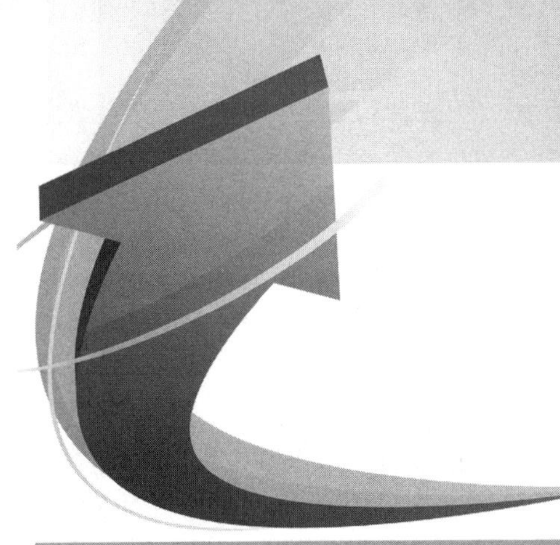

CASE 2.20
Bacteremia, Gram Negative | Level 3

SELF-ASSESSMENT ANSWERS

1. **Considering M. M.'s condition on admission and clinical course during this hospitalization, what organisms would be considered a likely potential cause of his infection when selecting empiric antimicrobial therapy?**

   Because M. M. has been hospitalized for 4 days in the ICU and has undergone abdominal surgery, he is at potential risk for infection from several organisms, including *Staphylococcus*, *Pseudomonas*, *Enterococcus*, *Klebsiella*, and others such as *Candida*, *Escherichia coli*, and *Enterobacter*.

2. **After reviewing the microbiology report revealing gram-negative bacteria from two sources, what would be an appropriate empiric therapy recommendation for this patient?**

   The development of an infection despite ongoing cefoxitin therapy would indicate the organism is resistant to this agent. Based on the nosocomial nature of this GNB infection, a dual-agent antipseudomonal regimen is warranted. Evolving extended-spectrum beta-lactamases (ESBLs) are not only resistant to penicillins, monobactams, cephalosporins, and cephamycins, they are also not affected by commercially available beta-lactamase inhibitors. Because the organism responsible for this infection may be ESBL+, the use of any penicillin or cephalosporin would not be advised. Vancomycin is not active against gram-negative bacterium. The patient has been receiving cefoxitin. Cephalosporins/cephamycins are more likely to induce ESBL-producing organisms, so a regimen containing a carbapenem and a second agent with antipseudomonal activity, like imipenem with tobramycin, would be recommended.

3. **Because the patient has had a splenectomy, which vaccine-preventable disease is he at a higher risk for contracting?**

   Patients that have had splenectomies are at a higher risk for developing infections with encapsulated organisms like pneumococci, *Haemophilus influenzae,* and meningococci. The CDC recommends that patients without a spleen receive these vaccines.

4. What would be an appropriate dose of once-daily gentamicin for this patient?

Although a gentamicin dose of 7 mg/kg is probably optimal for the treatment of infections due to *Pseudomonas*, doses of 4 to 7 mg/kg of ideal body weight have been discussed in the literature.

5. An M4 medical student is on trauma rotations this month, and she asks what the rationale is for dosing aminoglycosides once daily in patients that can tolerate it. You respond with a brief discussion about the pharmacodynamics of aminoglycosides. Which pharmacodynamic parameter best describes the rationale for dosing aminoglycosides once daily?

The pharmacokinetics parameter that governs aminoglycosides is C_{max}/MIC. The rationale behind dosing these drugs once daily is that with a larger dose, you can achieve a C_{max}/MIC ratio of greater than 8 to 10:1, which has been shown to increase bacterial killing and suppress the development of resistance.

6. One of M. M.'s blood cultures is positive for *Candida glabrata*, and the on-call resident asks you for an antifungal recommendation to treat this candidemia. Which of the following should you recommend?

a. Amphotericin B deoxycholate 3 mg/kg IV daily

b. Fluconazole 400-mg IV loading dose, then 200 mg IV daily

c. Terbinafine 250 mg IV daily

d. Caspofungin 70-mg IV loading dose, then 50 mg IV daily

e. Posaconazole 200 mg po tid

Answer d is correct. Choice a is incorrect. Amphotericin deoxycholate dosing for documented systemic candidiasis is 0.5 to 1 mg/kg daily, with a maximum daily dose of 1.5 mg/kg. Choice b is incorrect. *C. glabrata* is often resistant to fluconazole, and the recommended fluconazole dose for candidemia is 12 mg/kg or a loading dose of 800 mg, followed by a daily dose of 6 mg/kg or 400 mg. Choice c is incorrect. Terbinafine is not available for IV administration in the United States and is not recommended for systemic candidiasis. Choice d is correct. The 2009 IDSA *Clinical Practice Guidelines for the Management of Candidiasis* recommends fluconazole or an echinocandin for nonneutropenic candidemia. Because *C. glabrata* tends to be fluconazole resistant, an echinocandin would be recommended. Choice e is incorrect. Posaconazole 200 mg po tid is used for the prophylaxis for *Aspergillus* and/or candidemia in high-risk patients. This would not be recommended to treat candidemia.

BIBLIOGRAPHY

Moore RD, Lietman PS, Smith CR. Clinical response to aminoglycoside therapy: importance of the ratio of peak concentration to minimal inhibitory concentration. *J Infect Dis.* 1987;155(1):93-9.

Pappas PG, Kauffman CA, Andes D, et al; Infectious Diseases Society of America. Clinical practice guidelines for the management of candidiasis: 2009 update by the Infectious Diseases Society of America. *Clin Infect Dis.* 2009;48(5):503-35.

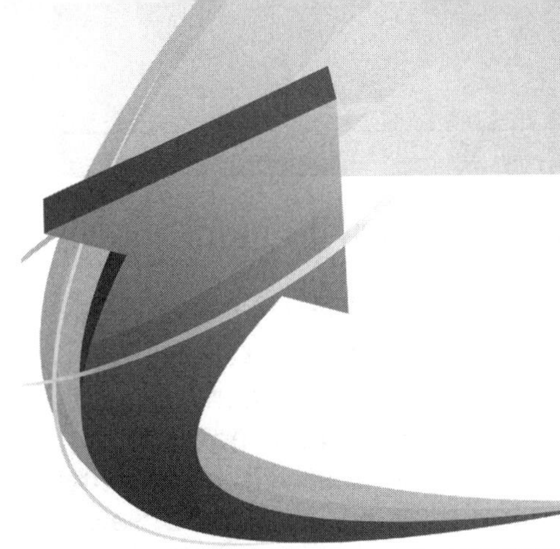

CASE 2.21
Severe Sepsis | Level 3

SELF-ASSESSMENT ANSWERS

1. **Describe the pathophysiology of severe sepsis.**

Severe sepsis is a complex disease process that involves inflammation, coagulation, and impaired fibrinolysis. Bacterial endotoxin and exotoxins initiate an inflammatory process involving the release of TNF-alpha and interleukins in addition to other pro-inflammatory cytokines. The release of the inflammatory cytokines damages endothelial cells and causes a release of tissue factor. Tissue factor subsequently activates the clotting process, resulting in the production of thrombin and reduced levels of protein C. The production of thrombin causes a down regulation in the enzyme thrombomodulin, which is responsible for activation of protein C. Finally, inflammation causes an increase rather than a decrease in the production of plasminogen activator inhibitor (PAI-1), which inactivates endogenous tissue plasminogen inhibitor, resulting in an impairment of fibrinolysis.

2. **On rounds in the ICU, the medical team asks you for your recommendations on whether J. J. should be placed on steroids for treating severe sepsis. What is your response?**

Randomized controlled trials using moderate doses of corticosteroids (hydrocortisone 200 IVPB mg/day, continuous infusion) have shown a reduction in mortality in patients' refractory to fluid replacement and vasopressor therapy. This is true particularly in patients with relative adrenal insufficiency. As a result, the 2012 sepsis and septic shock guidelines recommend the use of corticosteroids in patients who remain in septic shock despite adequate fluid replacement and vasopressor therapy. Steroids are not recommended if the patient is not in shock.

3. **The attending physician informs you that J. J.'s lactate level is 5.5 mmol/L. She asks you for your opinion on initial resuscitation goals for this patient. Based on the 2012 sepsis and septic shock guidelines, what is your response?**

The 2012 sepsis and septic shock guidelines recommend targeting initial resuscitation to normalize lactate in patients with elevated lactate levels (greater than or equal to 4.0 mmol/L). Additional goals during the first 6 hours of resuscitation include central venous pressure 8 to 12 mm Hg, mean arterial pressure greater than or equal to 65 mm Hg, urine output greater than or equal to 0.5 mL/kg/hr, and superior vena cava oxygenation saturation ($ScvO_2$) or mixed oxygen saturation (SvO_2) of 70% or 65%, respectively. This was based on a randomized, controlled study, which demonstrated that early goal-directed therapy could reduce the 28-day mortality rate.

4. According to the 2012 sepsis and septic shock guidelines, what would be the best initial fluid resuscitation regimen (fluid type and amount) for J. J.?

The 2012 sepsis and septic shock guidelines recommend that crystalloids be used as the initial fluid of choice in the resuscitation of severe sepsis and septic shock. The recommended initial fluid challenge in patients with sepsis-induced tissue hypoperfusion with suspicion of hypovolemia is to achieve a minimum of 30 mL/kg of crystalloids (a portion may be albumin equivalent). Thus, in the 80-kg patient, the best choice for initial fluid challenge would be 30 mL/kg × 80 kg = 2,400 mL of normal saline.

5. It is postulated that J. J.'s myocardial infarction may have been a result of sepsis-induced hypotension. How is the treatment of her severe sepsis impacted by her myocardial infarction?

According to the 2012 sepsis and septic shock guidelines, once tissue hypoperfusion has resolved and in the absence of extenuating circumstances, such as myocardial ischemia, severe hypoxemia, acute hemorrhage, or ischemic coronary artery disease, a red blood cell transfusion should occur when the hemoglobin concentration decreases to less than 7.0 g/dL to a target hemoglobin concentration of 7.0 to 9.0 g/dL. Red blood cell transfusions in septic patients can increase oxygen delivery. J. J. is not a candidate for a transfusion based on her myocardial infarction. Additionally, the use of erythropoietin as a specific treatment for anemia associated with severe sepsis is not recommended.

6. J. J.'s culture result from the bronchoscopy wash comes back reporting 4+ group A *Streptococcus*. Her antibiotics are changed from ceftriaxone to penicillin G 2 million units IVPB every 6 hours and clindamycin 900 mg IVPB every 8 hours. What is the rationale for using clindamycin in this situation, and what is an appropriate duration of antibiotic therapy?

The rationale for using clindamycin in combination with beta-lactam antibiotics, such as penicillin, in streptococcal and staphylococcal toxic shock syndromes comes from laboratory evidence, suggesting the clindamycin may suppress the production of bacterial toxin. Penicillins may be less effective against higher bacterial loads as some bacteria will enter a nonreplicative state and, therefore, decrease the activity of penicillins. This in vitro effect is called the *Eagle effect*. The addition of clindamycin or other protein synthesis inhibitors, such as linezolid, serve to suppress the formation of toxins and assist in eradicating the bacterial pathogen.

The duration of antibiotic therapy is 7 to 10 days for an immunocompetent patient. If a fungal infection is identified, therapy can be administered for 10 to 14 days. However, patients with a slow clinical response or those immunocompetent may require longer durations of therapy.

BIBLIOGRAPHY

Coyle EA; Society of Infectious Diseases Pharmacists. Targeting bacterial virulence: the role of protein synthesis inhibitors in severe infections. Insights from the Society of Infectious Diseases Pharmacists. *Pharmacotherapy.* 2003;23(5):638-42.

Dellinger RP, Levy MM, Rhodes A, et al; Surviving Sepsis Campaign Guidelines Committee including the Pediatric Subgroup. Surviving sepsis campaign: international guidelines for management of severe sepsis and septic shock: 2012. *Crit Care Med.* 2013;41(2):580-637.

Rivers E, Nguyen B, Havstad S, et al; Early Goal-Directed Therapy Collaborative Group. Early goal-directed therapy in the treatment of severe sepsis and septic shock. *N Engl J Med.* 2001;345(19):1368-77.

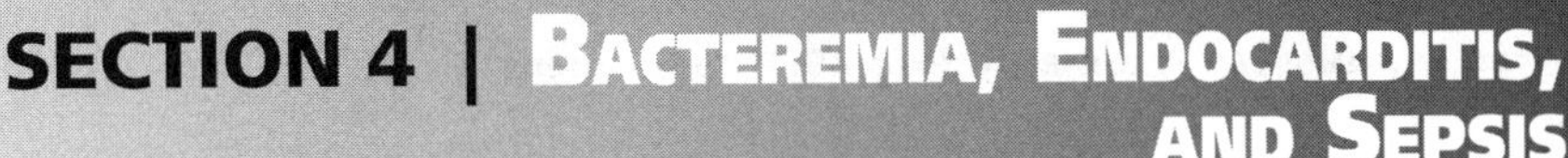

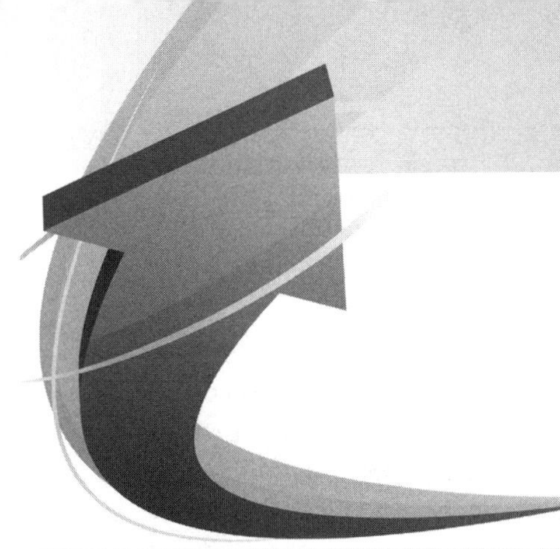

CASE 2.22
Septic Shock | Level 3

SELF-ASSESSMENT ANSWERS

1. **Based on the 2012 sepsis and septic shock guidelines for early goal-directed therapy, what is the most appropriate treatment plan at this time for J. S.?**

J. S. is currently hypotensive; therefore, there is an immediate need to try and elevate her blood pressure. Vasopressors are an option; however, prior to implementing vasopressors, it reasonable to try and maximize the CVP. Current guidelines recommend volume replacement as the initial step in trying to reverse the hypotension. Therefore, administration of IV fluids should continue in order to push the CVP into the range of 8 to 12 mm Hg prior to implementing vasopressor therapy. The recommended initial fluid challenge in patients with sepsis-induced tissue hypoperfusion with suspicion of hypovolemia is to achieve a minimum of 30 mL/kg of crystalloids (a portion may be albumin equivalent). If fluid replacement is unsuccessful in increasing the blood pressure, then vasopressors such as norepinephrine are the next option. High-dose steroids have not been shown to be beneficial in sepsis; indeed, recent meta-analyses have suggested that they may be harmful. Randomized controlled trials using moderate doses of corticosteroids (hydrocortisone 200 IVPB mg/day, continuous infusion) have shown a reduction in mortality in patients' refractory to fluid replacement and vasopressor therapy. This is true particularly in patients with relative adrenal insufficiency. As a result, the 2012 sepsis and septic shock guidelines recommend the use of corticosteroids in patients who remain in septic shock despite adequate fluid replacement and vasopressor therapy. A hydrocortisone taper is recommended once vasopressors are no longer required in the patient.

2. **Appropriate antimicrobial therapy continues to play a prominent role in the treatment of severe sepsis. Pharmacists can significantly impact outcomes from sepsis through their appropriate use. According to the 2012 sepsis and septic shock guidelines, appropriate antimicrobial therapy should be initiated within what time frame after recognition of septic shock?**

Although the initial focus for resuscitation of patients with severe sepsis should be focused on normalization of hemodynamic parameters, quick initiation of appropriate antimicrobial therapy is still an important component for optimal outcomes. Appropriate antimicrobial therapy should be initiated within the first hour of recognition of severe sepsis. Antimicrobial administration within the first hour of documented hypotension in septic shock was associated with increased survival. However, there is a 7.6% decrease in survival with every hour delay of antimicrobial treatment in these patients.

3. When should de-escalation to the most appropriate single agent be done after culture and sensitivity data are reported?

The 2012 sepsis and septic shock guidelines recommend that combination therapy in patients with severe sepsis should not be administered for longer than 3 to 5 days. Evidence from adequately powered, randomized clinical trials is not available to support combination over monotherapy other than in septic patients at high risk of death. There is no benefit of combination therapy once an organism is identified.

4. What are ways that an antimicrobial stewardship team could benefit the care of J. S.?

There are several ways that an antimicrobial stewardship team could benefit the care of this patient. First, the team can evaluate current antibiotics and make needed recommendations/changes due to patient characteristics (renal function, weight, etc). The team will also evaluate the appropriate use of antibiotics and respective pathogens, especially if cultures grow a resistant pathogen. The team can assist in streamlining antibiotics, changing to oral antibiotics when needed and monitor antibiotic efficacy and safety parameters. There is a mortality benefit for patients with severe sepsis and septic shock if empiric antimicrobials are de-escalated. Globally, antimicrobial stewardship programs can improve antibiotic and antifungal use and patient outcomes while decreasing pathogen resistance.

5. In evaluating whether to use normal saline or albumin for the fluid resuscitation in J. S., the medical team asks you for your recommendations. Based on your analysis of the literature, what should your response be?

The 2012 sepsis and septic shock guidelines support a high-grade recommendation for the use of crystalloids solutions in the initial resuscitation of patients with severe sepsis and septic shock. Current randomized controlled trials show no clear benefit in general of colloids over crystalloids; thus, crystalloids should be used from a cost effectiveness standpoint.

6. After fluid resuscitation, J. S. has the following hemodynamic parameters: mean arterial pressure 55 mm Hg, CVP 10 mm Hg, and cardiac index 3.0 L/min/m^2. The decision is made to administer a vasopressor. According to the 2012 sepsis and septic shock guidelines, what is the first choice therapy to administer in J. S.?

J. S.'s current hemodynamic parameters show an adequate cardiac index (normal 2.5 to 4.2) and central venous pressure (goal 8 to 12 mm Hg), but a low mean arterial pressure (goal equal to or greater than 65 mm Hg). Therefore, vasopressor therapy should be directed primarily at improving the blood pressure rather than enhancing inotropic support. The 2012 sepsis and septic shock guidelines list norepinephrine as the first line option for initiation of vasopressor support in patients with a normal or high cardiac index and a low mean arterial pressure. If J. S. had a low cardiac output, then inotropic support with the use of dobutamine may have been indicated.

BIBLIOGRAPHY

Dellinger RP, Levy MM, Rhodes A, et al; Surviving Sepsis Campaign Guidelines Committee including the Pediatric Subgroup. Surviving sepsis campaign: international guidelines for management of severe sepsis and septic shock: 2012. *Crit Care Med.* 2013;41(2):580-637.

Garnacho-Montero J, Gutiérrez-Pizarraya A, Escoresca-Ortega A, et al. De-escalation of empirical therapy is associated with lower mortality in patients with severe sepsis and septic shock. *Intensive Care Med.* 2014;40(1):32-40.

Kumar A, Roberts D, Wood KE, et al. Duration of hypotension before initiation of effective antimicrobial therapy is the critical determinant of survival in human septic shock. *Crit Care Med.* 2006;34(6):1589-96.

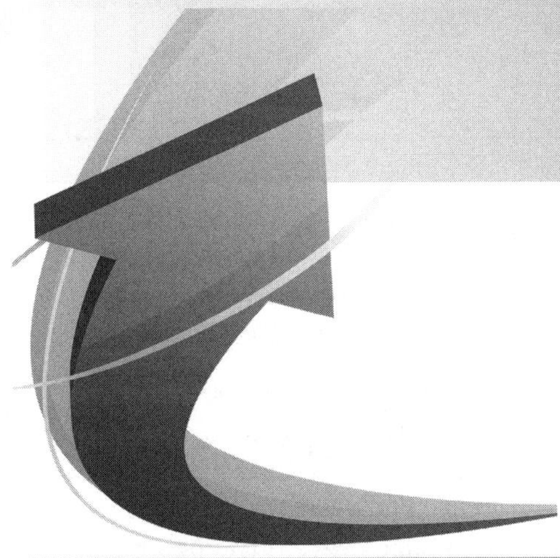

CASE 2.23
Complicated Urinary Tract Infection—Geriatric | Level 1

SELF-ASSESSMENT ANSWERS

1. What risk factors contribute to the development of a complicated UTI in J. M., and what potential pathogens could result in the complicated UTI/urosepsis in J. M.?

There are a number of risk factors that may contribute to the development of UTIs, including female gender, age, pregnancy, spermicide and/or diaphragm use, urinary catheter use, structural or functional abnormalities of the urinary tract, and the presence of neurologic dysfunction. The most frequent cause of complicated UTIs in male patients is instrumentation of the urinary tract, including the use of intermittent or indwelling urinary catheters or by undergoing a procedure such as a transurethral resection of the prostate. Urinary catheters increase the risk of infection by altering normal host defenses and promoting access of uropathogens into the bladder. As men age, the most frequent cause of infection is bladder obstruction due to benign prostatic hypertrophy (BPH). Urinary tract obstruction may lead to incomplete bladder emptying and may inhibit the normal flow of urine, disrupting the natural removal of bacteria from the bladder. This patient was admitted with a urinary catheter in place and has a past medical history significant for a stroke with residual hemiparesis and BPH, which may both contribute to incomplete bladder emptying and the development of UTIs.

The bacterial etiology of complicated UTIs, such as urosepsis and pyelonephritis, is more variable than uncomplicated UTIs due to the numerous factors that may contribute to their development (e.g., previous antibiotic use, presence of obstruction, use of catheters, etc.). The common causative bacteria in complicated UTIs include *Escherichia coli* (most common, 50% of cases), *Klebsiella pneumoniae*, *Proteus mirabilis*, *Pseudomonas aeruginosa*, *Enterobacter* species, *Serratia marcescens*, other gram-negative bacteria, *Enterococcus faecalis*, and *Candida* species. Because the preliminary results from this patient's urine and blood cultures are revealing the presence of a gram-negative rod, the most likely causative organism is *E. coli*, *K. pneumoniae*, *P. mirabilis*, *P. aeruginosa*, or *Enterobacter* species.

2. Based on the initial Gram stain results from the urine and blood cultures, which of the following antibiotics is most appropriate for the empiric treatment of J. M.'s complicated UTI?

- **a. Cefepime IV**
- **b. Ertapenem IV**
- **c. Oral TMP/SMX DS**
- **d. Ampicillin IV**
- **e. Oral doxycycline**

Answer a is correct. Given the nature of his clinical presentation, aggressive management with parenteral antimicrobials is warranted, so that oral TMP/SMX (c) or doxycycline (e) are not the best empiric therapy options for initial treatment in this patient. And, based on his clinical presentation and residence in a skilled nursing facility, empiric antibiotic therapy should provide coverage against potentially resistant gram-negative bacteria, including *P. aeruginosa*. Therefore, parenteral ampicillin (d) and ertapenem (b) would not be appropriate choices for this patient because they are inactive against *P. aeruginosa*. The patient is also allergic to penicillin antibiotics, providing further support against the use of ampicillin. Therefore, the most appropriate empiric antibiotic for this patient is parenteral cefepime (a), due to its excellent activity against gram-negative bacteria including *P. aeruginosa*. This patient has a history of developing a rash to penicillin but appears to have received cephalosporins (IM ceftriaxone) in the past without reaction.

3. The following day, the patient's fever and mental status improved, and the results of the urine and blood cultures and susceptibility results yield *Escherichia coli* susceptible to TMP/SMX, ampicillin/sulbactam, piperacillin/tazobactam, cefazolin, ceftriaxone, cefepime, imipenem, meropenem, levofloxacin, and tobramycin. Which of the following antibiotic regimens should be used for the continued treatment of J. M.'s infection (as directed therapy)?

- **a. Cefepime 2 g IVPB q 24 hr**
- **b. Meropenem 1 g IVPB q 12 hr**
- **c. Cefazolin 1 g IVPB q 12 hr**
- **d. Tobramycin 400 mg IVPB q 24 hr**
- **e. Aztreonam 1 g IVPB q 8 hr**

Answer c is correct. The results of the patient's urine and blood cultures reveal the presence of *E. coli,* which is susceptible to a number of different antimicrobials. Although the clinician could consider maintaining the patient on cefepime therapy, it is prudent to switch the patient to an antimicrobial that offers more directed coverage against the infecting bacteria (streamline or direct antimicrobial therapy against the infecting pathogen) to limit the effect of the broad-spectrum antibiotic on the patient's normal flora as well as to decrease the emergence of resistance. Because the infecting organism is susceptible to numerous antibiotics, cefepime (a), meropenem (b), aztreonam (e), and tobramycin (d) are not necessary to treat this patient's infection as they are fairly broad-spectrum agents with antipseudomonal activity. The dose listed for tobramycin is too high for the patient's level of renal function, and it is a potential nephrotoxic agent. Therefore, parenteral cefazolin (c) would be the most appropriate choice for continued antibiotic therapy in this patient due to its low cost and fairly narrow, directed spectrum of activity. It can be used parenterally until the patient stabilizes, at which time he can be converted to oral fluoroquinolone therapy for the remaining duration for his infection.

4. What is the recommended duration of antibiotic therapy for a patient with a complicated UTI, such as urosepsis and/or pyelonephritis?

The recommended duration of therapy for the treatment of patients with complicated UTIs is 7 to 14 days, depending on the infection type and severity of infection. Patients with infections such as pyelonephritis or urosepsis (especially with concomitant documented bacteremia) are typically treated for a total duration of 14 days, which can include both intravenous and oral therapy.

5. **Which of the following statements regarding urinary catheter use is *false* with regard to the development of UTIs?**
   a. **Urinary catheters do not increase the risk of developing UTIs.**
   b. **Bacteria may be introduced directly into the bladder during catheterization of the urinary tract.**
   c. **The longer the patient has a urinary catheter, the greater the chance of developing a UTI.**
   d. **In patients with long-term urinary catheters who develop symptomatic UTIs, replacement of the urinary catheter may decrease the incidence of reinfection.**
   e. **Antibiotic prophylaxis is not recommended in patients with long-term indwelling catheters to prevent the development of UTIs because it may lead to the emergence of resistant bacteria.**

Answer a is correct. The use of urinary catheters is frequently associated with the development of infection in the urinary tract due to alterations in normal host defenses and introduction of bacteria into the bladder. Bacteria can be introduced into the bladder during catheterization, by ascending up the outside lumen of the catheter along the mucosal border, or intraluminally via a contaminated collecting tube or drainage bag (b). The longer the patient has a urinary catheter, the greater the risk of developing a UTI (c). In patients with long-term (greater than 2 weeks) urinary catheters who develop symptomatic UTIs, the urinary catheter should be replaced to facilitate the resolution of symptoms and decrease the incidence of reinfection (d). Last, routine antibiotic prophylaxis is not recommended in patients with short-term or long-term indwelling urinary catheters to prevent the development of UTIs because they may postpone the development of bacteriuria and lead to the emergence of resistant bacteria (e).

6. **Which of the following pharmacologic and nonpharmacologic measures can be recommended in the prevention and management of UTIs in J. M.?**
   a. **Cranberry juice has been conclusively shown to decrease the incidence of UTIs in males.**
   b. **Phenazopyridine should be recommended to all patients with UTIs to provide symptomatic relief of pain and burning on urination.**
   c. **The use of a condom catheter or intermittent bladder catheterization should be considered in males who require urinary catheterization to decrease the rate of UTIs.**
   d. **Prophylactic antibiotic therapy, given systemically or by bladder irrigation, should be routinely administered during urinary catheter insertion to decrease the risk of catheter-associated UTIs.**
   e. **Long-term suppressive antibiotic therapy should be given to all patients with recurrent UTIs to decrease the occurrence of future UTIs.**

Answer c is correct. There are a number of pharmacologic and nonpharmacologic measures that can be offered to males who develop recurrent UTIs. Although cranberry juice may help decrease the occurrence of UTIs in some patients through its antioxidant and antibiotic effect, there is a lack of conclusive evidence on the therapeutic benefits of cranberry juice for the prevention of UTIs (a). Urinary analgesics, such as phenazopyridine, are used by some clinicians to alleviate the pain and burning associated with a UTI (b). However, many patients experience symptomatic relief soon after the initiation of antibiotic therapy so that urinary analgesics are not necessary. In addition, urinary analgesics may mask the symptoms of a UTI that is not responding to antibiotic therapy. In men for whom a urinary catheter is indicated and who have minimal postvoid residual urine, condom catheterization should be considered as an alternative to long-term indwelling catheterization to reduce the rate of catheter-associated bacteriuria and subsequent infection (c). Intermittent bladder catheterization should be considered as an alternative to long-term indwelling catheterization in patients with significant postvoid residual to reduce the incidence of catheter-associated bacteriuria and subsequent infection. The routine use of prophylactic antimicrobials (d), given systemically or by bladder irrigation, at the time of urinary catheter placement as a measure to decrease the rate of catheter-associated UTIs is not recommended at this time because there are insufficient data supporting its use. Lastly, long-term suppressive antibiotic therapy (e) is appropriate in certain patients with recurrent UTIs (recurrent UTIs without apparent precipitating events) but is not routinely recommended in all patients with recurrent UTIs due to the concern of the emergence of bacterial resistance.

BIBLIOGRAPHY

Hooton TM, Bradley SF, Cardenas DD, et al; Infectious Diseases Society of America. Diagnosis, prevention, and treatment of catheter-associated urinary tract infection in adults: 2009 International Clinical Practice Guidelines from the Infectious Diseases Society of America. *Clin Infect Dis.* 2010;50(5):625-63.

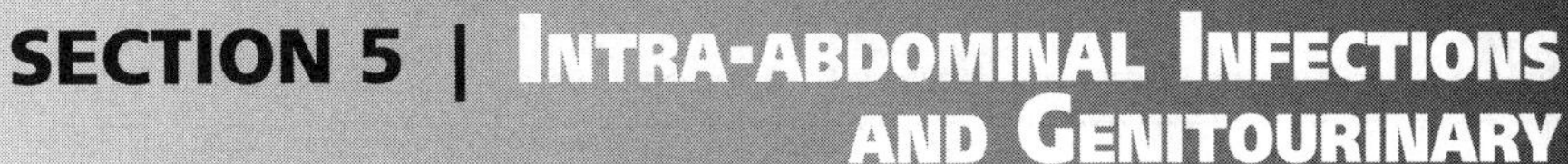

CASE 2.24
Urinary Tract Infection—Pediatric | Level 1

SELF-ASSESSMENT ANSWERS

1. **What is a risk factor for M. W. developing a UTI due to an extended-spectrum beta-lactamase-producing (ESBL) organism? What organisms, other than *Escherichia coli*, are likely to produce an ESBL?**

A recent history of antibiotic use is often strongly associated with emergence of resistant organisms. Several studies have suggested that patients with a history of cephalosporin and/or fluoroquinolone use are at increased risk for acquiring ESBL infections. *E. coli*, *Klebsiella*, and *Proteus* species are all known to produce ESBLs. The Clinical Laboratory and Standards Institute Subcommittee on Antimicrobial Susceptibility Testing has developed standards for detecting ESBLs in these organisms. Gram-positive organisms (e.g., streptococci, staphylococci, enterococci) and atypical organisms (e.g., *Legionella*, *Chlamydia*, *Mycoplasma*) do not produce ESBLs. Also, non-Enterobacteriaceae such as *Acinetobacter*, *Pseudomonas*, and *Stenotrophomonas* are usually multidrug resistant but are not typical ESBL-producers.

2. **According to the antibiogram, what is the likelihood that the organism causing M. W.'s UTI is resistant to amoxicillin?**

The correct answer is 45% because the numbers in the antibiogram represent the percentage of isolates susceptible to specific antimicrobials. *E. coli* is growing in M. W.'s urine culture and is the most common cause of UTIs. *E. coli* can become resistant to penicillins by producing a penicillinase. According to the antibiogram, 55% of *E. coli* isolates were susceptible to ampicillin; thus, 45% were resistant.

3. **According to the antibiogram, there is a 30% likelihood that the organism causing M. W.'s UTI ________.**

   a. **Produces an extended-spectrum beta-lactamase**
   b. **Has mutations in the folate synthesis enzymes**
   c. **Has a mutation in the 30S ribosomal subunit**
   d. **Produces an aminoglycoside-modifying enzyme**
   e. **Produces a fluoroquinolone efflux pump**

Answer b is correct. The numbers in the antibiogram represent the percentage of isolates susceptible to specific antimicrobials. *E. coli* is growing in M. W.'s urine culture and is the most common cause of UTIs. According to the antibiogram, 70% of *E. coli* were susceptible to TMP/SMX. Thus, 30% were resistant. TMP/SMX exerts antimicrobial activity by inhibiting enzymes in the bacterial folate synthesis pathway. Thus, mutation of bacterial folate synthesis enzymes would cause TMP/SMX resistance.

4. Why should imipenem/cilastatin be avoided for use in M. W.?

Beta-lactam antimicrobials have been associated with seizures, with carbapenems having a higher risk. Specifically, Primaxin® (imipenem/cilastatin) is known to cause seizures when used at high doses in patients with kidney impairment. Although M. W. has normal kidney function, Primaxin® should still be used with caution due to M. W.'s seizure disorder.

5. According to the antibiogram, what is the likelihood that the organism causing M. W.'s UTI is resistant to ceftriaxone?

The correct answer is 10% because the numbers in the antibiogram represent the percentage of isolates susceptible to specific antimicrobials. *E. coli* is growing in M. W.'s urine culture and is the most common cause of UTIs. According to the antibiogram, 90% of *E. coli* isolates were susceptible to cefotaxime—a third-generation cephalosporin. Thus, at least 10% were resistant. Ceftriaxone is also a third-generation cephalosporin and will likely have similar susceptibility to cefotaxime.

6. The hospital antibiogram can be used to ________.

a. Select antibiotic therapy after culture and susceptibilities have returned

b. Track the use of broad-spectrum antibiotics in a healthcare system

c. Monitor trends in antimicrobial resistance patterns over time

d. Guide empiric antiviral therapy during influenza season

e. Calculate the percentage of UTIs caused by *E. coli*.

Answer c is correct. Antibiotic susceptibility patterns can be monitored over time using annually or bi-annually published antibiograms. Choice a is incorrect because antibiograms guide empiric therapy and not pathogen-directed therapy after culture and susceptibilities return. Choice b is incorrect because antibiotic usage is not represented in antibiogram data. Choice d is incorrect because antiviral susceptibility testing is not usually depicted in antibiograms. Choice e is incorrect because the organisms represented come from all sources of infection (e.g., urine cultures, blood cultures, etc.).

BIBLIOGRAPHY

Bush K. Bench-to-bedside review: the role of beta-lactamases in antibiotic-resistant gram-negative infections. *Crit Care.* 2010;14(3):224.

Granowitz EV, Brown RB. Antibiotic adverse reactions and drug interactions. *Crit Care Clin.* 2008;24(2):421-42.

Montini G, Tullus K, Hewitt I. Febrile urinary tract infections in children. *N Engl J Med.* 2011;365(3):239-50.

Pakyz AL. The utility of hospital antibiograms as tools for guiding empiric therapy and tracking resistance. Insights from the Society of Infectious Diseases Pharmacists. *Pharmacotherapy.* 2007;27(9):1306-12.

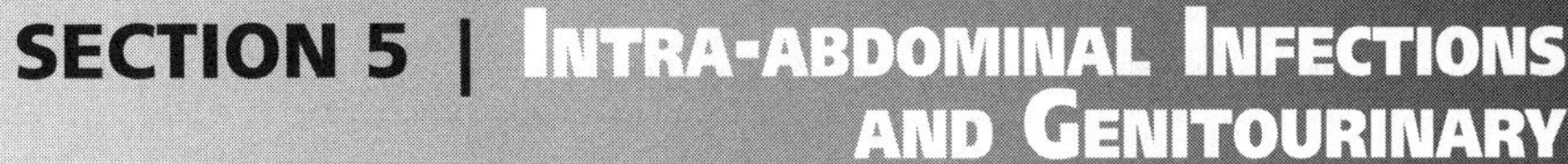

CASE 2.25
Uncomplicated Urinary Tract Infection | Level 2

SELF-ASSESSMENT ANSWERS

1. What are known risk factors for the development of a UTI? What symptoms, physical exam findings, and laboratory findings are suggestive of acute uncomplicated cystitis in this patient? What bacteria is the most common cause of acute uncomplicated cystitis in females?

There are a number of risk factors that may contribute to the development of UTIs, including female gender, age, pregnancy, spermicide and/or diaphragm use, and structural or functional abnormalities of the urinary tract. Urinary tract obstruction may lead to incomplete bladder emptying and inhibit the normal flow of urine, disrupting the natural removal of bacteria from the bladder. Females are at increased risk for the development of UTIs due to anatomical reasons (a short urethra that is in close proximity to the perianal area), which may promote bacterial colonization of the urethra and subsequent infection. Sexual intercourse promotes the entry of bacteria into the urinary bladder of females, where the bacteria may multiply and lead to a UTI. Urinary tract instrumentation may lead to bacterial colonization of the urinary bladder and subsequent UTI.

The presence of WBCs in the urine (pyuria) greater than 5 to 10 cells/hpf is suggestive of infection in the presence of symptoms compatible with a UTI. The most common signs and symptoms of a lower UTI include pain and burning on urination, increased urinary frequency and urgency, and suprapubic tenderness. A positive urinary nitrite occurs when gram-negative bacteria present in the urine metabolize dietary nitrates to nitrite. The urine specific gravity of 1.020 is normal and is not suggestive of a UTI.

Bacteria that cause acute uncomplicated cystitis in females typically originate from the bowel flora, which subsequently colonize the patient's urethra. Therefore, the most common cause of acute uncomplicated cystitis in females is *Escherichia coli,* which is responsible for approximately 80% to 90% cases of community-acquired UTIs. Other potential causative organisms associated with uncomplicated UTIs include *Proteus mirabilis, Klebsiella pneumoniae, Staphylococcus saprophyticus,* and *Enterococcus faecalis*. Organisms such as *Pseudomonas aeruginosa, Klebsiella oxytoca, Candida albicans*, and *Staphylococcus aureus* are rare causes of community-acquired UTIs but may be encountered as causative pathogens in complicated or hospital-acquired UTIs.

2. Which of the following pharmacologic and nonpharmacologic measures can be recommended in the management of UTIs in K. A.?

a. Cranberry juice has been conclusively shown to decrease the incidence of UTIs in females.

b. Phenazopyridine should be recommended to all patients with UTIs to provide symptomatic relief of pain and burning on urination.

c. In women who experience repeated symptomatic UTIs associated with sexual activity, voiding after intercourse may help prevent infection.

d. The use of spermicide-coated condoms during sexual intercourse may decrease the occurrence of UTIs.

e. Long-term suppressive antibiotic therapy should be given to all patients with recurrent UTIs to decrease the occurrence of future UTIs.

Answer c is correct. There are a number of pharmacologic and nonpharmacologic measures that can be offered to patients who develop recurrent UTIs. In young females who develop UTIs in association with sexual intercourse, voiding after intercourse will decrease the risk of infection by eliminating bacteria that may have been introduced into the bladder during intercourse. In addition, the use of spermicide-coated condoms during sexual intercourse increases *E. coli* growth in the vaginal tract, which may be introduced into the bladder during sexual intercourse and cause subsequent infection (d). Although cranberry juice may help decrease the occurrence of UTIs in some patients through its antioxidant and antibiotic effect, there is a lack of conclusive evidence on the therapeutic benefits of cranberry juice for the prevention of UTIs (a). Urinary analgesics, such as phenazopyridine, are used by some clinicians to alleviate the pain and burning associated with a UTI (b). However, many patients experience symptomatic relief soon after the initiation of antibiotic therapy so that urinary analgesics are not necessary. In addition, urinary analgesics may mask the symptoms of a UTI that is not responding to antibiotic therapy. Lastly, long-term suppressive antibiotic therapy (e) is appropriate in certain patients with recurrent UTIs (recurrent UTIs without apparent precipitating events) but is not routinely recommended in all patients with recurrent UTIs due to the concern of the emergence of bacterial resistance.

3. A first-year medical resident asks you for a recommendation regarding the appropriate antibiotic treatment for this patient's acute uncomplicated cystitis. The clinic outpatient antibiogram demonstrates that 82% of *Escherichia coli* isolates are susceptible to TMP/SMX. Which of the following regimens would be most appropriate to treat this patient's UTI?

a. Amoxicillin 500 mg po q 8 hr for 7 days

b. Azithromycin 1 g po as a single dose

c. Tetracycline 250 mg po q 6 hr for 7 days

d. TMP/SMX 1 DS tablet po bid for 3 days

e. Levofloxacin 250 mg po daily for 7 days

Answer d is correct. TMP/SMX for 3 days is the regimen of choice for the empiric treatment of acute uncomplicated cystitis in females in areas where local resistance rates of uropathogens do not exceed 20% (d). Therefore, because the TMP/SMX resistance rate to *E. coli* is 13%, TMP/SMX would be the most appropriate antibiotic to treat this patient's acute uncomplicated cystitis. Nitrofurantoin monohydrate/macrocrystals (100 mg twice daily for 5 days) or fosfomycin trometamol (3 g in a single dose) are also appropriate first-line options. Amoxicillin (a), tetracyclines (c), and azithromycin (b) are not considered useful agents for the treatment of UTIs due to their limited antibacterial activity against *E. coli* (high resistance rates) and the poor penetration of tetracycline and azithromycin into the urinary tract. In addition, our patient has an allergy to amoxicillin. Oral fluoroquinolones (e) are considered second-line treatment options for patients with acute uncomplicated cystitis due to their broad spectrum of activity and potential for collateral damage. A 7- to 10-day course of antibiotic therapy is no longer necessary for the treatment of acute uncomplicated cystitis because studies have demonstrated that a 3- to 5-day course of treatment is as effective as a 10-day regimen. Short-course therapy is not recommended in patients who have had previous infections caused by resistant bacteria, in male patients, or in patients with complicated UTIs.

4. If the results of the patient's urine hCG had been positive, which antibiotic class should not be used in any trimester during pregnancy because of potential harm to the unborn fetus?

The fluoroquinolones are pregnancy category C and should be avoided in pregnant patients because of potential fetal toxicity. The use of fluoroquinolones during pregnancy has been associated with arthropathy and cartilaginous damage in early toxicology studies in immature dogs. Therefore, fluoroquinolones should be given only during pregnancy if the benefits clearly outweigh the risks (patient has an infection due to an organism resistant to other potential alternatives). Trimethoprim should be avoided in the first trimester due to major congenital malformations, and sulfamethoxazole should be avoided in the third trimester due to bilirubin displacement. Tetracyclines should be avoided in pregnancy due to concerns of fetal teeth discoloration.

5. What antibiotic would be most appropriate to treat a nonpregnant female patient with acute uncomplicated cystitis who is allergic to sulfonamide antibiotics?

a. **Ceftriaxone 1 g IV daily**
b. **Doxycycline 100 mg po bid**
c. **Ciprofloxacin 250 mg po bid**
d. **Nitrofurantoin monohydrate/macrocrystals 100 mg po bid**
e. **Azithromycin 1 g po as a single dose**

Answer d is correct. TMP/SMX is the drug of choice for the empiric treatment of acute uncomplicated cystitis, except in patients allergic to sulfonamide antibiotics and in geographical areas where *E. coli* resistance rates to TMP/SMX exceed 20%. If this patient had an allergy to sulfonamide antibiotics, then oral nitrofurantoin monohydrate/macrocrystals 100 mg po bid × 5 days would be the recommended therapy (d). Doxycycline (b) and azithromycin (e) are not considered useful agents for the treatment of UTIs due to their limited antibacterial activity against *E. coli* and poor penetration into the urinary tract. Oral fluoroquinolones (c), such as ciprofloxacin, are considered second-line treatment options for patients with acute uncomplicated cystitis due to their broad spectrum of activity and potential for collateral damage. IV ceftriaxone (a) is not necessary for the treatment of this patient's acute uncomplicated cystitis due to its route of administration and need for IV access and the availability of alternative oral treatment options in this patient.

6. K. A. returns to the ambulatory clinic several months later with signs and symptoms of another episode of acute uncomplicated cystitis. Which of the following treatment strategies would be most appropriate for this patient?

a. **The current infection is most likely due to a resistant organism so the patient should be treated with a 14-day course of an oral fluoroquinolone, such as levofloxacin.**
b. **The current infection is most likely due to reinfection and should be treated with a 14-day course of TMP/SMX.**
c. **Due to K. A.'s frequent occurrences of UTIs (three episodes within 1 year), she should be treated for this episode of acute uncomplicated cystitis with TMP/SMX DS 1 tablet po bid for 3 days and counseled about lifestyle modifications in an attempt to decrease the recurrence of infection.**
d. **The patient should receive a 10-day course of IV ceftriaxone 1 g IV daily because oral therapy has been ineffective in the treatment of her infections.**

e. The patient's birth control should be switched to spermicide-coated condoms to minimize the development of recurrent UTIs.

Answer c is correct. The majority of recurrent infections are caused by reinfection, which is the recurrence of an infection by an organism different than the bacteria causing the preceding infection. Reinfections can often be treated with the same antibiotic that was used for the initial episode. Although this patient has had recurrent infections, it is not likely, at this point, that she has an infection due to a resistant organism requiring a different antibiotic (a fluoroquinolone [a] or ceftriaxone [d]). In addition, a longer course of TMP/SMX is also not necessary unless it is determined that this patient has a complicated UTI (b). The use of spermicide-coated condoms would not be useful in this patient because they increase the risk for the development of UTIs due to their effects on the protective vaginal flora, such as *Lactobacillus* (e). However, because the patient has experienced three UTIs in the past year and is experiencing acute symptoms, she should receive a prescription for TMP/SMX DS po bid × 3 days (she may receive TMP/SMX because it has been more than 3 months since last use) and receive counseling regarding the importance of lifestyle modification to prevent further episodes (e.g., void after sexual intercourse, wipe front to back after using the bathroom, avoid prolonged bathing, empty the bladder routinely during the day, maintain adequate hydration, avoid the use of spermicides, etc.) (c).

BIBLIOGRAPHY

Gupta K, Hooton TM, Naber KG, et al; Infectious Diseases Society of America; European Society for Microbiology and Infectious Diseases. International clinical practice guidelines for the treatment of acute uncomplicated cystitis and pyelonephritis in women: a 2010 update by the Infectious Diseases Society of America and the European Society for Microbiology and Infectious Diseases. *Clin Infect Dis.* 2011;52(5):e103-20.

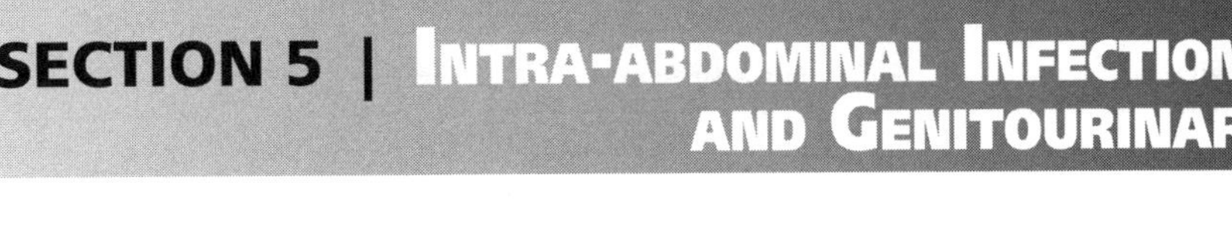

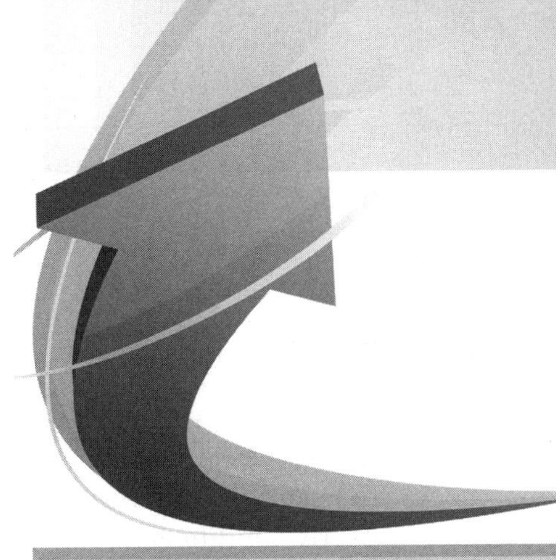

CASE 2.26
Intra-abdominal Infection | Level 3

SELF-ASSESSMENT ANSWERS

1. What is the optimal time frame in which antibiotics should be administered to a patient with an intra-abdominal infection?

Antimicrobial therapy should be administered based on an intra-abdominal infection diagnosis or when an intra-abdominal infection is suspected. For patients with hemodynamic and organ stability, antibiotics should be administered within 8 hours of presentation. In patients with septic shock, guidelines recommend the administration of antibiotics as soon as possible within the first hour.

2. The medical resident asks you if blood cultures should be ordered and drawn to identify the potential pathogen in P. H. What is the best response to the resident?

Blood cultures are rarely useful for diagnosing intra-abdominal infections and thus are not routinely recommended. In patients with community-acquired intra-abdominal infections, cultures do not provide additional relevant information. Studies demonstrate a low correlation of bacteremia to the identified pathogen in the abdominal infection. Bacteremia may be more common in patients admitted to the ICU or who are immunocompromised; thus, Gram stains and/or blood cultures may be beneficial in these situations. Because P. H. does not meet these characteristics, blood cultures would not be warranted at this time.

3. What recommendations would you make, if any, for the empiric antibiotic regimen that has been initiated for P. H.?

Empiric antimicrobial regimen options for community-acquired intra-abdominal infections are divided into mild-to-moderate infections and severe infections (determined by clinical judgment) as well as single agent and combination therapy. Mild-to-moderate infections can be treated with single agents such as cefoxitin, ertapenem, or moxifloxacin. Combination therapy includes cefazolin, cefuroxime, ceftriaxone, ciprofloxacin, or levofloxacin with metronidazole. For patients with severe infections, single agent options include imipenem/cilastatin, meropenem, doripenem, or piperacillin/tazobactam. Combination therapy includes cefepime, ceftazidime, ciprofloxacin, or levofloxacin with metronidazole. Antibiograms can assist with guiding therapy for patients. In P. H., the physician could have selected piperacillin/tazobactam or ertapenem as a single agent without the additional anaerobic coverage from metronidazole or could have opted for a cephalosporin or fluoroquinolone with metronidazole. Double coverage of anaerobes with piperacillin/tazobactam and metronidazole is not indicated in this situation; thus, therapy should be changed.

4. What if the physician had initiated levofloxacin and metronidazole for empiric therapy for P. H.? What recommendations would you make, if any, for the antibiotic regimen?

Based on this local antibiogram, fluoroquinolone resistant *Escherichia coli* exists. The IDSA intra-abdominal infection guidelines recommend that fluoroquinolones should be used only when hospital data show greater than 90% susceptibility data of *E. coli* to fluoroquinolones. Based on the severity of the infection and the antibiogram, cefepime or ceftriaxone could be alternatives for levofloxacin. Cefazolin and cefuroxime could be considered, but their susceptibilities are lower than cefepime or ceftriaxone. Imipenem, ertapenem, or piperacillin/tazobactam could be considered if single agent use were preferred.

5. What treatment duration is best to recommend for P. H.?

Duration of treatment for P. H. should be 4 to 7 days. If she had experienced uncomplicated diverticulitis, no antimicrobials would have been warranted.

6. You have been asked to participate in the new antimicrobial stewardship program at the hospital. Per the IDSA guidelines, what strategies could the program consider to initiate based on hospital resources?

Numerous strategies exist for antimicrobial stewardship programs in hospitals. The two core strategies are prospective audits of antimicrobial use with intervention and feedback to the prescriber and formulary restriction and preauthorization. The IDSA guidelines recommend programs also consider the following activities: education of the prescriber, development of clinical guidelines and pathways, antimicrobial order forms, de-escalation of therapy, dose optimization, and parental to oral conversion plans. Insufficient data exist to recommend antimicrobial cycling or combination therapy for preventing or reducing antimicrobial resistance.

BIBLIOGRAPHY

Dellit TH, Owens RC, McGowan JE Jr, et al; Infectious Diseases Society of America; Society for Healthcare Epidemiology of America. Infectious Diseases Society of America and the Society for Healthcare Epidemiology of America guidelines for developing an institutional program to enhance antimicrobial stewardship. *Clin Infect Dis.* 2007;44(2):59-77.

Solomkin JS, Mazuski JE, Bradley JS, et al. Diagnosis and management of complicated intra-abdominal infection in adults and children: guidelines by the Surgical Infection Society and the Infectious Diseases Society of America. *Clin Infect Dis.* 2010;50(2):133-64.

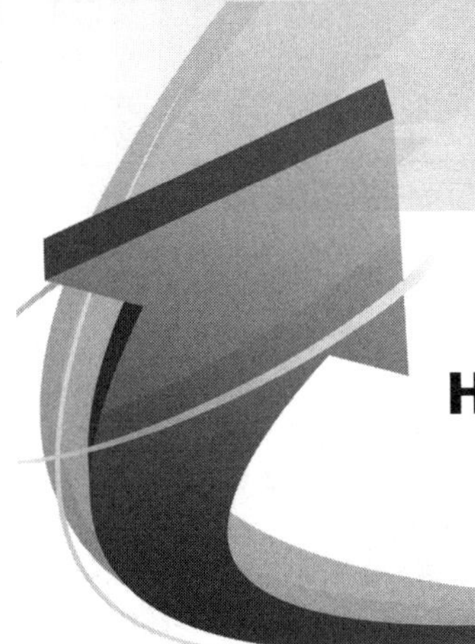

CASE 2.27

HIV—*Pneumocystis jirovecii* Pneumonia | Level 2

SELF-ASSESSMENT ANSWERS

1. **The physician wants to start sulfamethoxazole/trimethoprim. What is the best treatment regimen for J. C.?**

   Sulfamethoxazole/trimethoprim is dosed based on the trimethoprim component. The dose for the treatment of PCP in an HIV-positive patient is 15 to 20 mg/kg/day based on total body weight divided into three to four doses in the absence of renal insufficiency for 21 days.

2. **What alternative regimen for the treatment of PCP may result in hemolysis if administered to a patient with glucose-6-phosphate dehydrogenase deficiency?**

   Clindamycin and primaquine (oral), oral atovaquone, and IV pentamidine are alternatives to sulfamethoxazole/trimethoprim for the treatment of PCP according to the 2015 CDC opportunistic infections treatment guidelines. Primaquine is an oxidative drug that is contraindicated in the presence of glucose-6-phosphate dehydrogenase (G6PD) deficiency. IV pentamidine and oral atovaquone can be safely given in the presence of G6PD deficiency.

3. **What is the primary role of ritonavir in J. C.'s regimen?**

   Ritonavir is used as a "booster" in antiretroviral regimens. Although it is a protease inhibitor, ritonavir is no longer used at the therapeutic doses of 600 mg twice daily due to toxicities. Instead, it is used at low doses, typically 100 to 200 mg once or twice daily, to increase the serum concentration of other protease inhibitors, such as darunavir, which also delays the development of resistance.

4. **To deem the antiretroviral regimen a success, what should the plasma HIV RNA be at J. C.'s 2-month follow-up visit?**

   The goal of antiretroviral therapy is maximal and durable viral suppression to a plasma HIV RNA below the limits of detection, which vary with available community assays (e.g., less than 20 copies/mL commonly referred to as undetectable). According to the 2015 DHHS HIV treatment guidelines, at least a 1.0 log reduction from baseline is expected in the first 2 to 8 weeks after initiation of an antiretroviral regimen. Viral load is expected to be undetectable by weeks 8 to 24.

5. If J. C.'s work-up had revealed a PPD and a CXR consistent with active pulmonary tuberculosis, what antituberculous medication would be contraindicated with his antiretroviral regimen?

Protease inhibitors are metabolized through CYP3A4 and strong inhibitors of CYP3A4. Rifampin is a strong inducer of CYP3A4. When used in combination with rifampin, the serum concentration of protease inhibitors is significantly reduced, creating the likely potential for an ineffective regimen as well as resistance. A patient co-infected with HIV and TB should receive rifabutin in place of rifampin according to the 2003 American Thoracic Society TB guidelines and the 2015 CDC opportunistic infections treatment guidelines. There are no significant drug or dosing changes warranted when isoniazid, ethambutol, pyrazinamide, or pyridoxine are used in combination with protease inhibitors.

6. What is the most appropriate regimen for the prophylaxis of PCP, and how long should J. C. take it?

According to the guidelines, inhaled pentamidine, dapsone 100 mg daily, sulfamethoxazole/trimethoprim DS daily, and atovaquone 1,500 mg daily are indicated for the prophylaxis of PCP. Sulfamethoxazole/trimethoprim is the most preferred regimen. Dapsone and atovaquone are alternatives to sulfamethoxazole/trimethoprim. Clindamycin and primaquine is an alternative to sulfamethoxazole/trimethoprim for the treatment of PCP. Secondary prophylaxis (in patients who have had PCP) should be continued on therapy until their CD4 count is greater than or equal to 200 cells/mm^3 for 3 months as a result of immunologic response from antiretroviral therapy.

BIBLIOGRAPHY

American Thoracic Society; CDC; Infectious Diseases Society of America. Treatment of tuberculosis. *MMWR Recomm Rep.* 2003;52(RR-11):1-77.

Panel on Opportunistic Infections in HIV-Infected Adults and Adolescents. Guidelines for the Prevention and Treatment of Opportunistic Infections in HIV-Infected Adults and Adolescents: Recommendations from the Centers for Disease Control and Prevention, the National Institutes of Health, and the HIV Medicine Association of the Infectious Diseases Society of America. http://aidsinfo.nih.gov/contentfiles/lvguidelines/adult_oi.pdf. Accessed June 14, 2015.

Panel on Opportunistic Infections in HIV-Exposed and HIV-Infected Children. Guidelines for the Prevention and Treatment of Opportunistic Infections in HIV-Exposed and HIV-Infected Children. Department of Health and Human Services. http://aidsinfo.nih.gov/contentfiles/lvguidelines/oi_guidelines_pediatrics.pdf. Accessed February 21, 2015.

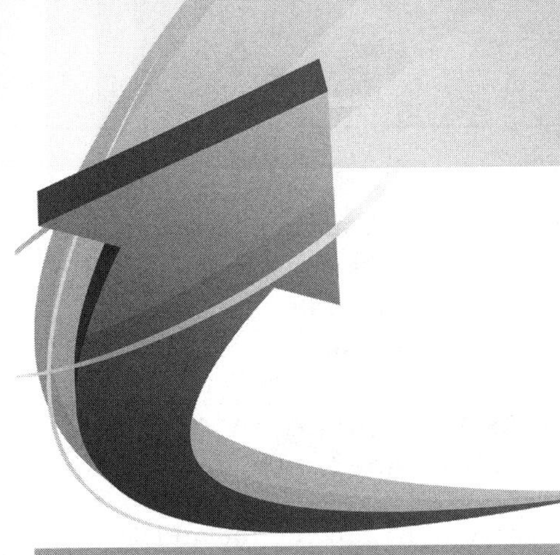

CASE 2.28
HIV Medication Management | Level 2

SELF-ASSESSMENT ANSWERS

1. What ART must be avoided for treatment of this patient's HIV? What ART remains as options for this patient?

The presence of the HLAB5701 allele increases the patient's risk of experiencing the abacavir systemic hypersensitivity reaction. Therefore, the use of abacavir is contraindicated. Although the patient has first-generation nonnucleoside resistance, etravirine is a second- or next-generation nonnucleoside reverse transcriptase inhibitor that is FDA-approved for use in treatment-experienced patients. It will still maintain its activity. The patient's virus is R5 tropic, so maraviroc, a CCR5 antagonist would be appropriate. It is FDA-approved for use in treatment-experienced patients. Boosted darunavir and atazanavir are protease inhibitors that are FDA-approved for use in protease-inhibitor naïve patients, so it would be an acceptable agent to use. Raltegravir, elvitegravir, and dolutegravir are integrase inhibitors that are FDA-approved for use in integrase-inhibitor susceptible patients.

2. What is the most appropriate recommendation for P. T.'s opportunistic infection prophylaxis plan?

Primary prophylaxis for *Pneumocystis jirovecii* pneumonia is recommended when CD4 counts are less than 200 cells/mm^3. This patient has a sulfa allergy, which makes first-line bactrim inappropriate. This patient also has G6PD deficiency, so second-line dapsone is inappropriate. Third-line agent atovaquone is appropriate for PCP prophylaxis because the CD4 is 180. Primary prophylaxis for *Mycobacterium avium* complex is indicated when CD4 counts are less than 50 cells/mm^3. Primary prophylaxis for toxoplasmosis is initiated when CD4 counts are less than 100 cells/mm^3 and toxoplasma IgG+. Primary prophylaxis of cryptococcal meningitis and cytomegalovirus retinitis is not indicated. These CD4 count recommendations and medications are per 2015 CDC opportunistic infections treatment and prevention guidelines.

3. What is the most appropriate therapy for HIV for P. T. at this time?

a. Change regimen to lamivudine, tenofovir, and efavirenz

b. Change regimen to zidovudine, lamivudine, and tenofovir

c. Change regimen to abacavir, lamivudine, darunavir, and ritonavir

d. Change regimen to tenofovir, emtricitabine, and dolutegravir

e. Change regimen to tenofovir, emtricitabine, and rilpivirine

Answer d is correct. The patient's genotype reveals resistance to first-generation nonnucleoside reverse transcriptase inhibitors (efavirenz and nevirapine). Thus, neither of these medications should be included as part of the regimen (a). The 2015 DHHS guidelines recommend the combination of three active medications for the treatment of HIV in an experienced patient. The use of a triple nucleoside reverse transcriptase inhibitor regimen like tenofovir, lamivudine, and zidovudine is not recommended (b). The use of abacavir is contraindicated in the presence of the HLAB5701 allele medications (c). Rilpivirine is FDA-indicated only in treatment-naïve patients and should be avoided if viral load is greater than 100,000 (e). The best choice is tenofovir, emtricitabine, and dolutegravir (d), which is a preferred regimen according to the 2015 DHHS guidelines in naïve patients and can be used in experienced patients susceptible to integrase inhibitors.

4. A patient initiating therapy with efavirenz should be informed of the potential for what adverse effect?

a. Jaundice

b. Vivid dreams

c. Skin hyperpigmentation

d. Lipodystrophy

e. Peripheral neuropathy

Answer b is correct. Jaundice (a) is associated with atazanavir. Skin hyperpigmentation (c) is associated with emtricitabine. Lipodystrophy (d) is associated with protease inhibitors and stavudine. Peripheral neuropathy (e) is associated with stavudine, didanosine, and zalcitabine. Vivid dreams (b) are associated with the nonnucleoside reverse transcriptase inhibitor efavirenz. In addition, efavirenz may cause severe depression, suicidal ideation, or nonfatal suicide attempts; thus, this patient should be counseled and followed up closely due to his history of depression.

5. What vaccines are appropriate to administer to P. T. at this time?

He should receive the Tdap vaccine and the HPV series. The pneumococcal vaccine is appropriate to administer to P. T.; however, PCV 13 should be administered first followed by PPSV 23 8 weeks later per the Advisory Committee on Immunization Practices. He should also receive the inactivate influenza vaccine yearly, as the live vaccine is contraindicated. Hepatitis A and B vaccines are inappropriate because the HAV and HBV surface antibodies are positive, indicating protection.

6. Patients should be counseled to administer all of the following antiretroviral agents with a meal except _______.

a. Rilpivirine

b. Efavirenz

c. Darunavir

d. Elvitegravir

e. Atazanavir

Answer b is correct. The absorption of efavirenz (b) is significantly increased in the presence of a high-fat food, which may result in an increased incidence of adverse effects. It should be administered on an empty stomach. Food significantly affects the increased absorption of rilpivirine and should be administered with at least 400 calories (a). Darunavir (c), atazanavir (e), and elvitegravir (d) should also be administered with food to improve absorption.

BIBLIOGRAPHY

Panel on Antiretroviral Guidelines for Adults and Adolescents. Guidelines for the use of antiretroviral agents in HIV-1-infected adults and adolescents. Department of Health and Human Services. http://aidsinfo.nih.gov/contentfiles/lvguidelines/AdultandAdolescentGL.pdf. Accessed June 15, 2015.

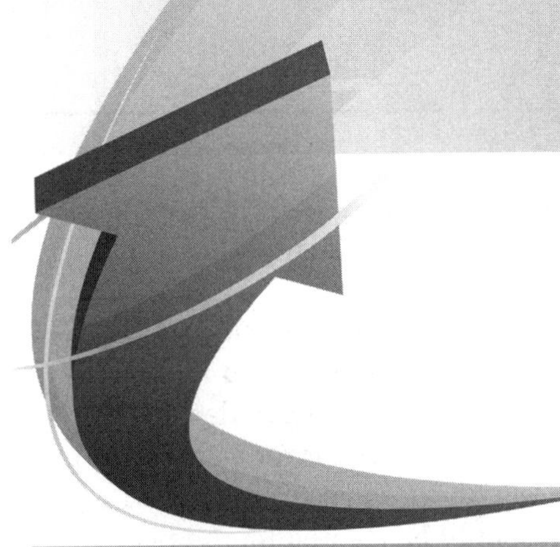

CASE 2.29
Vulvovaginal Candidiasis | Level 1

SELF-ASSESSMENT ANSWERS

1. **What is the most common cause of vulvovaginal candidiasis?**

   Candida albicans accounts for 80% to 90% of cases of vaginal candidiasis. The remainder of cases are caused by *Candida tropicalis* and *Candida glabrata* or other yeasts. *Gardnerella vaginalis* is a common cause of bacterial vaginosis. *Trichomonas vaginalis*, a protozoa, also is a cause of vaginosis, but vulvovaginal candidiasis is not a sexually transmitted disease.

2. **What are signs, symptoms, and risk factors of vulvovaginal candidiasis?**

   Common signs and symptoms of vaginal candidiasis include itching, burning, irritation, vaginal soreness, dyspareunia, nonodorous discharge that may be watery to thick, and erythema of the labia/vulva.

   Risk factors for vaginal candidiasis include pregnancy, use of broad-spectrum antibiotics, use of high estrogen-containing oral contraceptives, corticosteroids or other agents that are immunosuppressive, an immunosuppressed host (for reasons other than medications), diabetes mellitus (especially if poorly controlled), sexual activity (especially with use of a diaphragm), and poor hygiene.

3. **Over-the-counter (OTC) vaginal candidiasis products are appropriate for ________.**

   a. **Patients with similar symptoms who have had a previously diagnosed vaginal yeast infection**
   b. **Pregnant women**
   c. **Recurrent (more than four episodes per year) vaginal candidiasis**
   d. **Patients less than 12 years of age**
   e. **Patients with foul-smelling vaginal discharge**

   Answer a is correct. Over-the-counter products are recommended for individuals who have been previously diagnosed with vaginal candidiasis (a). Symptoms should be similar to past episodes as vaginal candidiasis may be mistaken for bacterial vaginosis or a sexually transmitted disease. A pregnant woman (b) should be referred to her physician for treatment of vaginal candidiasis. The CDC's *Sexually Transmitted Diseases Treatment Guidelines, 2015* recommend only the use of topical azole therapy for 7 days in pregnancy. Recurrent vaginal candidiasis (c) may indicate a more serious problem that needs to be evaluated by a physician. Recurrences may be secondary to HIV, uncontrolled diabetes, immunosuppression, oral contraceptives, or hormone replacement therapy. Patients less than 12 years of age (d) should be referred to a physician for diagnosis and treatment. Patients with foul-smelling vaginal discharge (e) should also be referred to a physician for appropriate diagnosis and treatment. Foul-smelling discharge likely represents a different diagnosis than vulvovaginal candidiasis (e.g., bacterial vaginosis).

4. What are appropriate drug therapy options (nonprescription and prescription) for vulvovaginal candidiasis? Compare and contrast these agents.

Miconazole, tioconazole, and clotrimazole are available as nonprescription topical agents. Terconazole, butoconazole, and fluconazole are available by prescription only. Topical nonprescription therapy is recommended for most patients as initial therapy. Fluconazole is available as an oral prescription only. (See the CDC's *Sexually Transmitted Diseases Treatment Guidelines, 2015*.)

From clinical trials for acute vaginal candidiasis, it appears that both oral and topical therapies are equally efficacious. Topical azole drugs are more effective than nystatin. Fluconazole is approved for the treatment of vaginal candidiasis as a single oral dose of 150 mg and is available only by prescription. Fluconazole may improve patient compliance as the topical preparations are recommended to be used for 3 to 7 days (although single-dose therapy can be used). Fluconazole is a generally more costly treatment option than the OTC topically administered products because a physician office visit is usually necessary to obtain a prescription.

5. What is the appropriate treatment duration for vulvovaginal candidiasis?

Depending on the drug and formulation, duration of treatments can be from 1 to 14 days in length. Short-course topical formulations can be used as a one-time dose or for 1 to 3 days in uncomplicated vulvovaginal candidiasis. Pregnant women should be treated for 7 days.

6. All of the following statements are appropriate counseling points for L. D. *except* ________.

- **a. Signs and symptoms should improve in 48 to 72 hours.**
- **b. Common adverse effects associated with intravaginal antifungal products include vulvovaginal irritation, burning, and pruritus.**
- **c. Complete the full course of therapy.**
- **d. Stop using the medication if menstruation begins.**
- **e. Certain products are oil-based and may weaken a latex condom or diaphragm.**

Answer d is correct. L. D. should continue using the topical antifungal preparation even if menstruation begins. She needs to complete the entire course of therapy even if symptoms subside prior to completing therapy (c). Symptoms should improve within 48 to 72 hours (a) and resolve within a week. If symptoms persist, she should contact her physician. It is important to advise L. D. that certain products are oil-based and may weaken latex condoms and diaphragms (e). If she uses latex condoms or a diaphragm for contraception, a non-oil-based product may be necessary. Common adverse effects associated with intravaginal antifungal products include vulvovaginal irritation, burning, and pruritus (b).

BIBLIOGRAPHY

Workowski KA, Bolan G; Centers for Disease Control and Prevention (CDC). Sexually transmitted diseases treatment guidelines, 2015. *MMWR Recomm Rep.* 2015;64(RR-03):1-137.

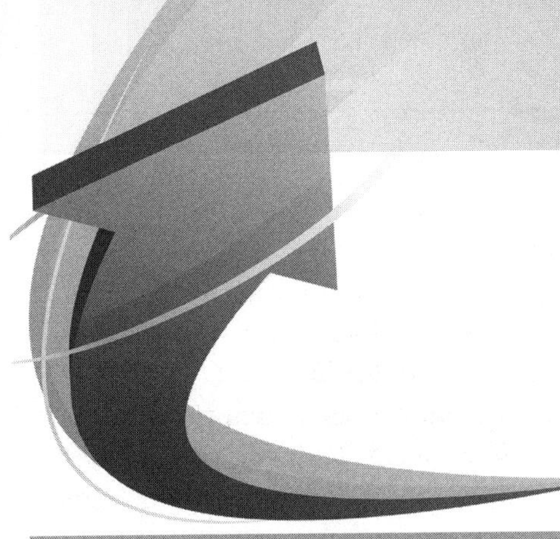

CASE 2.30
Disseminated Candidiasis | Level 3

SELF-ASSESSMENT ANSWERS

1. What are risk factors for disseminated (systemic) candidiasis? What are M. B.'s risk factors?

Risk factors for candidemia include total parenteral nutrition (TPN), central venous catheters, broad-spectrum antibiotic use, immunosuppression, neutropenia, abdominal surgery, mechanical ventilation, and being in the ICU (especially prolonged stays). Hospitalization alone is not a risk. Disseminated candidiasis is being considered in M. B. because she has had multiple abdominal surgeries, has been on broad-spectrum antibiotics, has had TPN, has a central venous catheter, and has been in the ICU for 15 days. Also, despite broad-spectrum antimicrobial therapy (vancomycin, meropenem, tobramycin), M. B. is critically ill. She also has yeast in her urine and sputum. Her blood cultures are negative × 2 days; however, the yield of a positive *Candida* blood culture is low (less than 50%). Often, disseminated candidiasis is a diagnosis of exclusion.

2. What is the most appropriate antifungal agent for M. B. at this time?

The IDSA's 2009 *Clinical Practice Guidelines for the Management of Candidiasis* recommend fluconazole or an echinocandin as initial therapy for most adults. The guidelines suggest an echinocandin in patients with moderately severe to severe illness or in those who have previously received an azole. M. B. has continued to clinically worsen despite receiving fluconazole for several days. Voriconazole is an option for candidiasis and has a broader spectrum of activity than fluconazole. However, because M. B. failed fluconazole therapy it may be prudent to avoid the empiric use of voriconazole as the potential for cross-resistance exists. Data demonstrate that voriconazole may not be appropriate therapy in refractory candidiasis in patients previously treated with fluconazole. Therefore, based on current guidelines, an echinocandin such as caspofungin, micafungin, or anidulafungin should be consider the most appropriate antifungal for M. B. at this time.

Some institutions report susceptibilities to fungal isolates, if available, knowing the prevalence of non-*albicans Candida* species may lead to selecting an echinocandin empirically.

3. Which species of *Candida* is intrinsically resistant to fluconazole?

Candida krusei is intrinsically resistant to fluconazole. Acquired resistance may occur with any of the other *Candida* species. For example, *C. glabrata* is frequently resistant to the azole class as a result of efflux pumps.

4. A physician asks you for a recommendation for antifungal therapy. Upon review of patient information, you notice that the patient has a creatinine clearance of 15 mL/min. Which agent should be avoided in this patient?

a. Liposomal amphotericin
b. Voriconazole oral
c. Anidulafungin IV
d. Voriconazole IV
e. Fluconazole oral

Answer d is correct. Intravenous administration of voriconazole (d) should be avoided in patients with a CrCl less than 50 mL/min due to accumulation of an excipient (cyclodextrin) in the IV formulation. Oral voriconazole (b) may be administered to a patient with a CrCl of 15 mL/min. Dosage adjustment for oral voriconazole is not required for patients with renal impairment. Dosage adjustment for fluconazole (e) is required for patients with renal impairment, but the agent may be administered to those with a CrCl of 15 mL/min. Dosage adjustment for renal impairment is not required for liposomal amphotericin (a) or anidulafungin (c).

5. What agents would be considered appropriate empiric therapy if a non-*albicans* *Candida* species was suspected?

Non-*albicans Candida* may be resistant to fluconazole, especially in critically ill patients. Echinocandins (micafungin, caspofungin, anidulafungin) have activity against all *Candida* species. Amphotericin B is also active against most commonly isolated species of *Candida* (resistance with *C. lusitaniae* and *C. guilliermondii*). Voriconazole is also appropriate for most *Candida* species (consider a different antifungal class if patient has had recent azole exposure).

6. What antifungals are active against *Aspergillus* species?

Aspergillus fumigatus is the most common species responsible for invasive aspergillosis. *Aspergillus flavus, Aspergillus niger*, and *Aspergillus terreus* are the next most common species. Caspofungin, amphotericin B, posaconazole, itraconazole, and voriconazole are active against *Aspergillus* species. Micafungin and anidulafungin have activity against *Aspergillus* species but are not FDA approved for this indication. Fluconazole is not active against *Aspergillus* species. Voriconazole is the recommended agent of choice for the primary treatment of invasive aspergillosis in most patients.

BIBLIOGRAPHY

Pappas PG, Kauffman CA, Andes D, et al; Infectious Diseases Society of America. Clinical practice guidelines for the management of candidiasis: 2009 update by the Infectious Diseases Society of America. *Clin Infect Dis.* 2009;48(5):503-35.

Walsh TJ, Anaissie EJ, Denning DW, et al; Infectious Diseases Society of America. Treatment of aspergillosis: clinical practice guidelines of the Infectious Diseases Society of America. *Clin Infect Dis.* 2008;46(3):327-60.

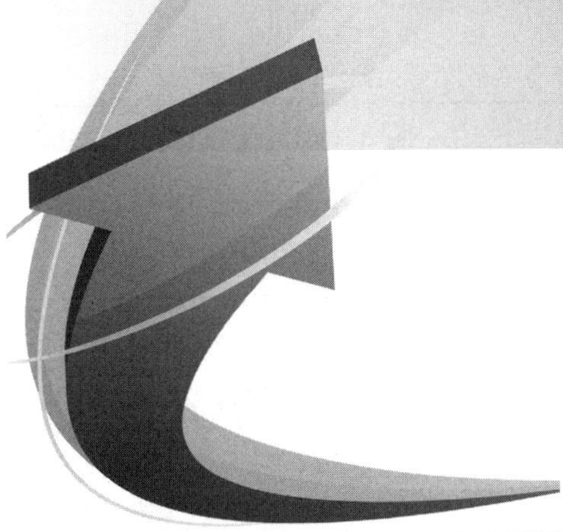

CASE 2.31
Lyme Disease | Level 1

SELF-ASSESSMENT ANSWERS

1. What main risk factors does S. H. have for developing Lyme disease?

Lyme disease prevalence has not been shown to differ between gender and age groups. Outdoor activities in wooded areas place people at risk for Lyme disease. People who infrequently go outdoors are less likely to be bitten by a tick and thus have a lower risk of acquiring Lyme disease. It is advisable to wear light-colored clothing when spending time outdoors to more easily see ticks on clothing so that they may be removed before attachment to skin occurs. In the United States, the Centers for Disease Control and Prevention has determined that endemic areas include nonurban communities throughout much of the Northeast (Massachusetts to Maryland), parts of the upper Midwest (Minnesota and Wisconsin), and areas along the West Coast (northern California and Oregon). Finally, patients who have removed a tick within 24 hours of attachment are at low risk of developing Lyme disease. It is not until a tick has been attached for greater than 36 hours that patients should be considered at highest risk for infection with *Borrelia burgdorferi*, the organism responsible for Lyme disease in the United States.

2. S. H.'s physical findings are most consistent with which stage of Lyme disease?

Signs and symptoms of early Lyme disease found on physical exam include erythema migrans as well as nonspecific symptoms such as low-grade fever, fatigue, malaise, lethargy, headache, myalgia, and arthralgia. Late Lyme disease occurs months after disease onset, and S. H. returned from camping 10 days ago. Late Lyme disease may present with rheumatologic (arthritis) and/or neurological manifestations (encephalomyelitis, peripheral neuropathy, or encephalopathy), which is also not consistent with S. H.'s physical exam. Lyme carditis is incorrect as S. H.'s heart rate is within normal limits and a physical exam revealed normal sinus rhythm. Lyme arthritis is a manifestation of late Lyme disease. Post Lyme-disease syndrome is categorized by chronic signs and symptoms of Lyme disease despite conventional antimicrobial management. S. H. has not yet received antimicrobial treatment.

3. **Which of S. H.'s lab results, besides ELISA, is most consistent with Lyme disease?**

Elevated ESR is a nonspecific indicator of inflammation that occurs in 50% of patients with erythema migrans. Platelets are typically normal in patients with Lyme disease. WBC count is usually normal or mildly elevated in Lyme disease.

4. **What would be the most appropriate treatment regimen for S. H., and what is the duration of treatment?**

S. H.'s Lyme disease is classified as early localized erythema migrans, which is treated using doxycycline 100 mg po bid, cefuroxime axetil 500 mg po bid, or amoxicillin 500 mg po tid. Azithromycin 500 mg po daily, rather than 250 mg po daily, may be used, although it has been shown to be somewhat less effective than doxycycline, cefuroxime, and amoxicillin for eradicating *B. burgdorferi*. Thus, azithromycin should be reserved for treatment of patients who cannot tolerate first-line agents. The IDSA's 2006 Lyme disease guidelines recommend a 10- to 21-day duration of treatment with doxycycline for patients with early uncomplicated Lyme disease. The duration of 14 to 21 days is recommended for amoxicillin or cefuroxime axetil.

5. **The most effective way for S. H. to prevent future episodes of Lyme disease would be ________.**

   a. **Ceftriaxone 1 g IM × 1 dose after prolonged outdoor activity**
   b. **Administration of the Lyme disease vaccine**
   c. **Application of tick repellent containing DEET to skin before outdoor activity**
   d. **Doxycycline 100 mg po bid during the summer months**
   e. **Azithromycin 1 g po weekly during the summer months**

Answer c is correct. The use of repellents such as DEET has been shown to prevent Lyme disease (c). No vaccine is currently available to prevent Lyme disease in humans (b). Early antibiotic prophylaxis may be used to prevent erythema migrans at the site of a tick bite but should not be used prior to exposure (a, d, e).

6. **What immunizations does S. H. need at this time?**

S. H. needs the Tdap vaccine and the annual influenza vaccine (if appropriate timing) at this time. She does not have risk factors to meet criteria for the hepatitis A or B, pneumococcal, or meningococcal vaccine. She is older than the age range for the HPV vaccine. The physician diagnosis of chicken pox excludes her from needing the varicella vaccine.

BIBLIOGRAPHY

Wormser GP, Dattwyle RJ, Shapiro ED, et al. The clinical assessment, treatment, and prevention of Lyme disease, human granulocytic anaplasmosis, and babesiosis: clinical practice guidelines by the Infectious Diseases Society of America. *Clin Infect Dis.* 2006;43(9):1089-134.

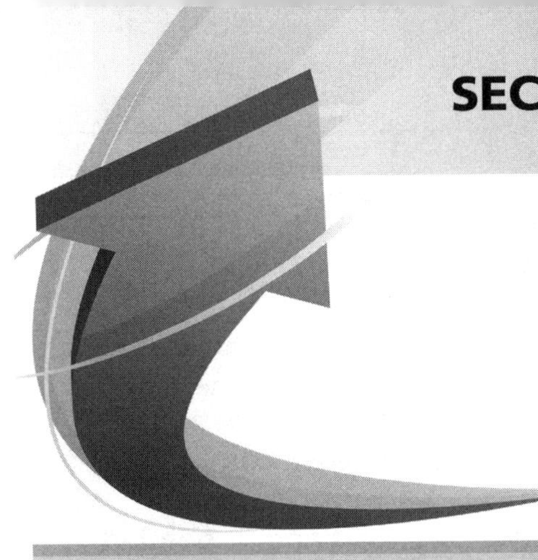

CASE 2.32
Neisseria gonorrhea | Level 2

SELF-ASSESSMENT ANSWERS

1. Empiric antimicrobial coverage should include agent(s) that are active against what organism(s)?

N. gonorrheae is a gram-negative diplococci. According to the CDC's 2015 STD treatment guidelines, individuals infected with gonococci are frequently co-infected with *Chlamydia trachomatis*; thus, patients should be treated with an antimicrobial regimen that provides coverage for both organisms. Typically, this is dual therapy.

2. What is the most appropriate treatment regimen for R. C.'s infection?

According to the CDC's 2015 STD treatment guidelines, a patient with gonorrhea should also be treated for chlamydia. A single 250-mg IM dose of ceftriaxone effectively treats *N. gonorrhea* but not *C. trachomatis*. If ceftriaxone is not available, a single 400-mg dose of cefixime may be used as an alternative, but it does not provide as high or sustained bactericidal blood levels as ceftriaxone. In addition, elevated MICs of cefixime have been noted, which may be the beginning of resistance. In 2007, the CDC cited an increasing incidence of fluoroquinolone-resistant gonorrhea, thus recommending that ciprofloxacin, levofloxacin, and other quinolones not be used for treatment. A single 1,000-g dose of azithromycin or 7-day course of doxycycline 100 mg po bid effectively eradicates *C. trachomatis* but not *N. gonorrhea*. Ceftriaxone 250 mg IM × 1 with azithromycin 1,000 mg orally × 1 will effectively treat both gonorrhea and chlamydia. It is recommended to administer both antimicrobial agents on the same day.

3. What are potential complications of untreated gonorrhea?

N. gonorrheae can cause infections of the cervix, urethra, rectum, or pharynx. Gonococcal conjunctivitis is uncommon. Potential complications from gonorrhea include pelvic inflammatory disease (PID) in women. Approximately 15% of women with gonorrhea develop PID. Disseminated gonorrhea can occur in females or males, but it is three times more likely to occur in women. Males can experience prostatitis, epididymitis, or inguinal lymphadenopathy from gonorrhea, but these are all rare complications.

4. How long should R. C. be counseled to abstain from sexual intercourse?

To minimize transmission, a patient with gonorrhea and/or chlamydia should abstain from intercourse for 7 days following single-dose treatment or until a 7-day treatment regimen is completed and the patient is asymptomatic. All sexual partners (defined by the CDC as "persons having sexual contact with the infected patient within the 60 days preceding onset of symptoms or gonorrhea diagnosis") should be treated for both infections. If the last sexual encounter occurred greater than 60 days previously, the last partner should be treated. In addition, all patients diagnosed with gonorrhea should be tested for other STDs including HIV and syphilis.

5. If R. C. has been pregnant and had a history of an anaphylactic reaction to cephalexin, what is the most appropriate agent to empirically treat gonorrhea?

Ceftriaxone and azithromycin are appropriate agents for empiric treatment of gonorrhea and chlamydia in pregnant patients. Ceftriaxone is inappropriate to use in a patient with a history of anaphylaxis to a cephalosporin like cephalexin; thus, the 2015 guidelines recommend dual treatment with oral gemifloxacin 320 mg × 1 plus oral azithromycin 2 g × 1 or treatment with gentamicin 240 mg IM × 1 plus azithromycin 2 g orally × 1. However, fluoroquinolones, like ciprofloxacin, and tetracyclines, like doxycycline, are contraindicated in pregnancy; thus, consultation with an ID specialist is recommended in a pregnant patient with a cephalosporin allergy. Gonorrhea in pregnancy should be treated to prevent ophthalmia neonatorum.

6. If R. C. had presented with complaints of tender joints and arthritic symptoms, what would be the diagnosis and, if needed, what would be the recommended treatment regimen?

Tenosynovitis, monoarticular arthritis, and tender necrotic skin lesions are symptoms of a disseminated gonococcal infection. Treatment recommendations, per the CDC, are hospitalization of the patient and administration of ceftriaxone 1 g IM or IV daily for 7 days and azithromycin 1,000 mg orally × 1 dose. Cefotaxime is an alternate regimen to ceftriaxone dosed at 1 g IV every 8 hours. Although symptoms improve in a few days, 7 days of treatment is recommended. However, after 24 to 48 hours of improvement, therapy may be switched to the oral route based upon antimicrobial susceptibility testing.

BIBLIOGRAPHY

Workowski KA, Bolan G; Centers for Disease Control and Prevention (CDC). Sexually transmitted diseases treatment guidelines, 2015. *MMWR Recomm Rep.* 2015;64(RR-03):1-137.

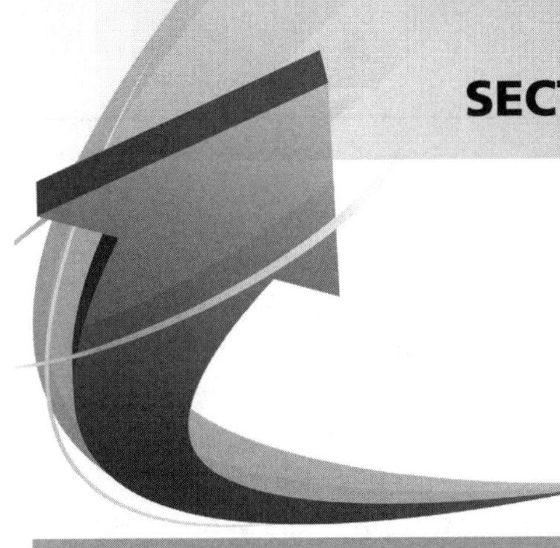

CASE 2.33
Genital Herpes | Level 3

SELF-ASSESSMENT ANSWERS

1. **What is an appropriate treatment regimen that could be effectively used to treat T. J.'s acute genital HSV episode?**

According to the CDC's 2015 STD treatment guidelines, the following regimens are recommended for a recurrent episode of genital HSV: acyclovir 400 mg po tid × 5 days, 800 mg po bid × 5 days or 800 mg po tid × 2 days, famciclovir 125 mg po bid × 5 days, 1,000 mg bid × 1 day or 500 mg once then 250 mg bid × 2 days, or valacyclovir 500 mg po bid × 3 days or 1 g po daily × 5 days. Valganciclovir is not recommended for the treatment of genital HSV. IV acyclovir is recommended for patients with severe disease or who require hospitalization for complications from HSV. Topical antiviral therapy has shown minimal benefit and is not recommended.

2. **The primary goal of treatment of recurrent episodes of HSV with acyclovir is which of the following?**

   a. **Eradication of HSV through cidal effects on the virus**
   b. **Symptomatic control through inhibition of viral replication**
   c. **Concomitant prevention of herpes zoster infections**
   d. **Management of bacterial superinfection caused by virus-induced tissue damage**
   e. **Prevent acquisition of sexually transmitted diseases other than HSV from an infected partner**

Answer b is correct. Treatment of recurrent genital HSV with acyclovir or any other currently marketed antiviral agent will not eradicate the virus (a). The goal of antiviral therapy in this setting is symptomatic control through inhibition of ongoing viral replication (b). Periodic short courses of acyclovir are unlikely to prevent herpes zoster infection (c). Although bacterial superinfection may be a complication of HSV infection, treatment with acyclovir will not manage bacterial superinfection, nor will acyclovir prevent the acquisition of other STDs (d, e).

3. **What therapy should be recommended for chronic suppressive therapy if T. J. began to experience greater than 10 episodes per year of genital HSV?**

Chronic suppressive regimens reduce the frequency of genital HSV recurrences by 70% to 80% in patients that experience greater than six episodes per year. Recommended suppressive regimens by the CDC include acyclovir 400 mg po twice daily, famciclovir 250 mg po twice daily, or valacyclovir 500 mg once daily or 1,000 mg once daily. Although valacyclovir is an acceptable therapeutic option for chronic suppressive therapy, the 500-mg daily dose has been shown to be somewhat less effective than the 1,000-mg daily dose or acyclovir in patients with very frequent exacerbations (10 or more episodes per year). Once-daily valacyclovir has been shown to reduce ~50% of HSV-2 transmissions within discordant, heterosexual couples. Famciclovir has been shown to be not as effective in suppressing viral shedding compared to acyclovir or valacyclovir.

4. Had T. J. been diagnosed HIV positive with severe, disseminated HSV infection, what would be the most appropriate treatment regimen to use?

Parenteral antiviral therapy is indicated in HIV-infected patients with severe or disseminated HSV infection. The parenteral form of acyclovir dosed at 5 to 10 mg/kg every 8 hours would be indicated in this setting. IV therapy is recommended for 2 to 7 days or until clinical improvement followed by oral therapy completing at least 10 total days of treatment. Ganciclovir IV, foscarnet IV, and valganciclovir have activity against HSV but are typically reserved for CMV treatment and are not preferred therapies for HSV infection. Oral acyclovir is relatively poorly absorbed and would not be expected to provide high enough systemic concentrations to effectively treat severe or disseminated HSV in immunocompromised hosts.

5. Which of the following counseling points is appropriate for T. J.?

a. Episodic therapy reduces the risk of transmission.

b. Sexual transmission occurs only during symptomatic periods.

c. Her sex partner(s) should not worry about being infected unless the partner(s) has/have symptoms.

d. It is not necessary for T. J. to inform current and future sex partners that she has genital herpes.

e. T. J. should abstain from sexual activity with uninfected partners when lesions or prodromal symptoms are present.

Answer e is correct. All persons with genital herpes should abstain from sexual activity with uninfected persons when lesions or prodromal symptoms are present (e). They should also be encouraged to inform current sex partners that they have genital herpes and inform future partners before beginning a sexual relationship (d). Episodic therapy does not reduce the risk of transmission of HSV (a), and sexual transmission of HSV can occur during asymptomatic periods (b). Sex partners of infected persons should be informed that they might be infected even if they are asymptomatic (c). Sex partners of patients with documented STDs should be referred to their physician for evaluation and possible treatment of that particular as well as other STDs.

6. T. J. becomes pregnant and has two recurrent episodes during pregnancy. The infant is born, and the pediatrician is concerned for disseminated neonatal herpes. What is the appropriate treatment regimen for the infant?

The case-fatality rate of neonatal herpes is approximately 50%. Of those who do survive, morbidity is high, and permanent neurological damage occurs frequently. In the situation where the mother has a history of herpes at term or acquired HSV during the first trimester, the incidence of transmitting HSV to the infant is very low at less than 1%. However, when a pregnant women acquires HSV near delivery (in the third trimester), the risk of transmission of HSV from the mother to infant is high (30% to 50%). In the postnatal period few cases occur, primarily from direct contact of an infected person with an acute lesion.

Because the pediatrician is concerned about HSV in the infant in this question, it is important to obtain cultures and initiate treatment in known or suspected infants with IV acyclovir dosed at 20 mg/kg every 8 hours. Infants with proven disseminated or CNS disease should be treated for 21 days with IV therapy. Infants with disease focused to the skin or mucous membranes may be treated for 14 days duration.

BIBLIOGRAPHY

Workowski KA, Bolan G; Centers for Disease Control and Prevention (CDC). Sexually transmitted diseases treatment guidelines, 2015. *MMWR Recomm Rep.* 2015;64(RR-03):1-137.

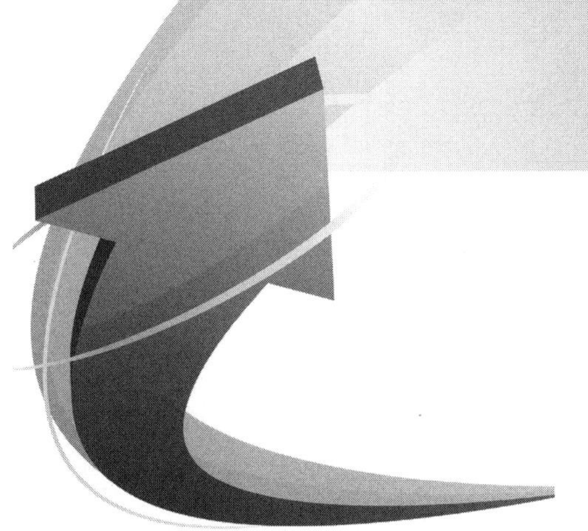

APPENDIX

APPENDIX: COMMON MEDICAL TERMINOLOGY AND ABBREVIATIONS

Abbreviation	Medical Terminology
A1c	Glycosylated hemoglobin
Abd	Abdomen
ACIP	Advisory Committee on Immunization Practices
AIDS	Acquired immunodeficiency syndrome
ALP	Alkaline phosphatase
ALT	Alanine transaminase
AOM	Acute otitis media
APGAR	Appearance, Pulse, Grimace, Activity, Respiration
ART	Antiretroviral therapy
ASHP	American Society of Health-System Pharmacists
AST	Aspartate aminotransferase
BCG	Bacillus Calmette–Guérin
bid	Two times daily
BP	Blood pressure
BPH	Benign prostatic hypertrophy
bpm	Beats per minute
BS	Bowel sounds
BUN	Blood urea nitrogen
CABG	Coronary artery bypass graft/grafting
CAD	Coronary artery disease
cap	Capillary
CA-MRSA	Community-associated methicillin-resistant *Staphylococcus aureus*
cART	Combination antiretroviral therapy
CBC	Complete blood count
CCE	Clubbing, cyanosis, or edema
CCR5	C-C chemokine receptor type 5
CD4	Cluster of differentiation 4 (a glycoprotein)
CDC	Centers for Disease Control and Prevention
CDI	*C. difficile* infection
CI	Cardiac index
CK	Creatine kinase
CKMB	MB isoenzyme of creatine kinase
CMV	Cytomegalovirus
CN	Cranial nerve
CNS	Central nervous system
CO	Cardiac output
CO_2	Carbon dioxide
COPD	Chronic obstructive pulmonary disease
CrCl	Creatinine clearance

Abbreviation	Medical Terminology
CRP	C-reactive protein
CSF	Cerebrospinal fluid
CT	Computerized tomography
CTA	Clear to auscultation
CTAB	Clear to auscultation bilaterally
CV	Cardiovascular
CVA	Cerebrovascular accident
CVAT	Costovertebral angle tenderness
CVP	Central venous pressure
CXR	Chest x-ray
D5LR	Dextrose 5% in lactated Ringer's (solution)
D5NS	Dextrose 5% in normal saline
D5W	Dextrose 5% in water
D10W	Dextrose 10% in water
D/C	Discontinue
DDD	Defined daily dose
DEET	N,N-diethyl-meta-toluamide
DFA	Direct fluorescent antibody
DHHS	Department of Health and Human Services
DNA	Deoxyribonucleic acid
DOT	Days of therapy
DS	Double strength
DTaP	Diphtheria, tetanus, and pertussis
ECG	Electrocardiogram
ED	Emergency department
EOM(I)	Extraocular muscles (intact)
ELISA	Enzyme-linked immunosorbent assay
EMS	Emergency medical services
Ext	Extremities
ESBL	Extended-spectrum beta-lactamase
ESR	Erythrocyte sedimentation rate
F	Farenheit
FBG	Fasting blood glucose
FDA	Food and Drug Administration
Fe	Iron
FiO_2	Fraction of inspired oxygen
FTA-ABS	Fluorescent treponemal antibody absorption
G6PD	Glucose-6-phosphate-dehydrogenase
GBS	Group B *Streptococcus*
GE	Gastroenteritis
GEN	General

APPENDIX (cont'd)

Abbreviation	Medical Terminology
GNB	Gram-negative bacilli
gtt	Drop
GU	Genitourinary
HAV	Hepatitis A virus
HBV	Hepatitis B virus
HCAP	Healthcare-associated pneumonia
hCG	Human chorionic gonadotropin
HCO_3	Bicarbonate
HEENT	Head, eyes, ears, nose, throat
HepA	Hepatitis A
HF	Heart failure
HFA	Hydrofluoroalkane
Hg	Hemoglobin
Hib	*Haemophilus influenzae* type b
HIV	Human immunodeficiency virus
HMG-CoA	3-hydroxy-3-methyl-glutaryl-CoA
hpf	High power field
HPV	Human papillomavirus
hr	Hour
HR	Heart rate
HSV	Herpes simplex virus
Ht	Height
HTN	Hypertension
ICU	Intensive care unit
ID	Infectious disease
IDSA	Infectious Diseases Society of America
IgE	Immunoglobulin E
IgG	Immunoglobulin G
IIV	Inactivated influenza vaccine
IM	Intramuscular
INH	Isoniazid
INR	International normalized ratio
IV	Intravenous
IVDA	Intravenous drug abuse
IVP	Intravenous push
IVPB	Intravenous piggyback
LAD	Lymphadenopathy
lb	Pound
KOH	Potassium hydroxide
LLL	Lower left lung
LMP	Last menstrual period

Abbreviation	Medical Terminology
LPF	Low power field
M4	Fourth-year medical student
MAO	Monoamine oxidase
MI	Myocardial infarction
min	Minute
MIC	Minimal inhibitory concentration
Micro	Microbiology
MMR	Measles, mumps, and rubella
m/r/g	Murmurs/rubs/gallops
MRSA	Methicillin-resistant *Staphylococcus aureus*
MS	Muscle strength
MSM	Men who have sex with men
MSSA	Methicillin-susceptible *Staphylococcus aureus*
MVA	Motor vehicle accident
MVI	Multivitamin
NAD	No abnormality detected; no apparent distress
NC/AT	Normocephalic/atraumatic
Neuro	Neurological
NKDA	No known drug allergies
NS	Normal saline
NSAID	Nonsteroidal anti-inflammatory drugs
NSR	Normal sinus rhythm
NTND	Nontender, nondistended
N/V/D	Nausea, vomiting, diarrhea
O_2 sat	Oxygen saturation
ODT	Orally disintegrating tablet
OP	Oropharynx
ORIF	Open reduction and internal fixation
OTC	Over-the-counter
OU	Both eyes (from Latin *oculi uterque*)
$PaCO_2$	Partial pressure of carbon dioxide in the blood
PAI-1	Plasminogen activator inhibitor-1
PaO_2	Partial pressure of oxygen in the blood
PBP	Penicillin-binding protein
pCO_2	Partial pressure of carbon dioxide
PCP	Primary care provider; *Pneumocystis* (*jirovecii*) pneumonia
PCV	Pneumococcal conjugate vaccine
PCWP	Pulmonary capillary wedge pressure
PERRLA	Pupils equally round and reactive to light and accommodation

APPENDIX (cont'd)

Abbreviation	Medical Terminology
pH	Potential of hydrogen
PID	Pelvic inflammatory disease
PMN	Polymorphonuclear neutrophil
po	By mouth, orally (from Latin *per os*)
pO_2	Partial pressure of oxygen
PPD	Purified protein derivative (tuberculin screening skin test)
PPSV	Pneumococcal polysaccharide vaccine
pr	Per rectum
prn	As needed (from Latin *pro re nata*)
PVC	Premature ventricular contraction
q	Every
qam	Every morning
QFT-GIT	QuantiFERON-TB Gold In-Tube test
qhs	Every night at bedtime (from Latin *hora somni)*
qid	Four times daily
qpm	Every evening
QTc	QT interval, corrected for heart rate
RA	Room air
RBC	Red blood cell
Rect	Rectal
RNA	Ribonucleic acid
ROM	Range of motion
rpm	Respirations per minute
RPR	Rapid plasma reagin
RR	Respiratory rate
RRR	Regular rate and rhythm
SC	Subcutaneous
$ScvO_2$	Superior vena cava oxygenation saturation
S/D/M	Systolic, diastolic, and mean (pressures)
sec	Second

Abbreviation	Medical Terminology
segs	Segmented cells
SIDP	Society of Infectious Diseases Pharmacists
SOB	Shortness of breath
SSRI	Selective serotonin reuptake inhibitor
STD	Sexually transmitted disease
SvO_2	Mixed venous oxygen saturation
SVR	Systemic vascular resistance
T_4	Thyroxine
T	Temperature
TB	Tuberculosis
Td	Tetanus, diphtheria
Tdap	Tetanus, diphtheria, and pertussis
TEE	Transesophageal echocardiogram
TIBC	Total iron-binding capacity
tid	Three times daily
TMP/SMX	Trimethoprim/sulfamethoxazole
TNF	Tumor necrosis factor
TPN	Total parenteral nutrition
TSH	Thyroid-stimulating hormone
tsp	Teaspoon
TTE	Transthoracic echocardiogram
UA	Urinalysis
UTI	Urinary tract infection
VAR	Varicella (chickenpox)
VDRL	Venereal Disease Research Laboratory (test)
VS	Vital signs
WBC	White blood cell
WD	Well developed
WDWN	Well developed, well nourished
WNL	Within normal limits
Wt	Weight

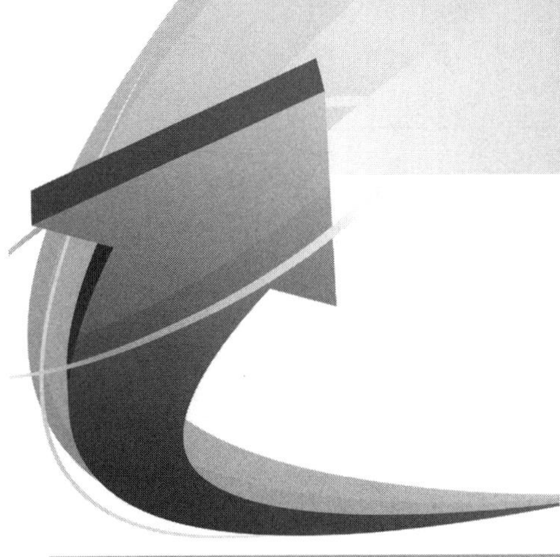

INDEX

A

D

E

F

G

H

I

J

L

M

T

U

V

Z